Praise for
THE SOUP CLEANSE

"Finally, a healthier way to detox! The nourishing recipes in THE SOUP CLEASE are a great foundational tool to optimize your wellness and encourage weight loss."

—Jen Widerstrom, fitness expert, TV personality,
and trainer on NBC's *The Biggest Loser*

"Your diet is a crucial part of sustaining positive mental health, and THE SOUP CLEANSE is an option that can help align your body and mind. I recommend THE SOUP CLEANSE as a refreshing alternative to typical juice-cleanse programs currently on the market."

—Dr. Charles Sophy, FACN, author of *Side by Side:
The Revolutionary Mother-Daughter Program
for Conflict-Free Communication*

"THE SOUP CLEANSE brings to the public this brilliant idea of using organic soups that are nutrient rich, yeast- and gluten-free, with a variety of colors and tastes for our patients with digestive compromise or weight-loss needs."

—Farshid Sam Rahbar, MD, ABIHM, holistic
and integrative gastroenterologist

THE SOUP
CLEANSE

A Revolutionary Detox of
Nourishing Soups *and* Healing Broths

Angela Blatteis *and*
Vivienne Vella

FOUNDERS OF SOUPURE

with *Rachel Holtzman*

Foreword by Nada Milosavljevic, MD, JD,
Director, Integrative Health Program,
Massachusetts General Hospital

GRAND CENTRAL
Life & Style
NEW YORK · BOSTON

Copyright © 2015 by Angela Blatteis and Vivienne Vella

Cover design by Lisa Forde
Cover photograph by Oscar Zagal
Cover copyright © 2017 by Hachette Book Group, Inc.

Grand Central Life & Style
Hachette Book Group
1290 Avenue of the Americas, New York, NY 10104
grandcentrallifeandstyle.com
twitter.com/grandcentralpub

Originally published in hardcover and ebook by Grand Central Life & Style in December 2015
First trade paperback edition: December 2017

Grand Central Life & Style is an imprint of Grand Central Publishing. The Grand Central Life & Style name and logo are trademarks of Hachette Book Group, Inc.

The publisher is not responsible for websites (or their content) that are not owned by the publisher.

The Hachette Speakers Bureau provides a wide range of authors for speaking events. To find out more, go to www.hachettespeakersbureau.com or call (866) 376-6591.

Photography by Victor Boghossian Photography, copyright © 2015
The "Dirty Dozen Plus" and "Clean Fifteen" mentioned on pages 48 and 49 are trademarks of the Environmental Working Group.

Library of Congress Control Number: 2015949895

ISBNs: 978-1-4555-9506-8 (trade paperback), 978-1-4555-3665-8 (ebook)

Printed in the United States of America

LSC-C

10 9 8 7 6 5 4 3 2 1

We dedicate this book to all busy, hardworking parents who are looking for better nutrition for themselves and their families. Anyone out there with tired eyes and blurred vision from reading tiny labels with ingredients you don't recognize—we dedicate this to you too. To those suffering from injuries or recovering from surgeries, we offer this book to you in the hope that our bone broths and soups help heal your bodies and bring you the comfort only a good bowl of soup can provide.

We come onto this earth with one body. It is our temple, and we must nurture it to thrive and feel our best. Whether you have come to realize the importance of good nutrition through research, education, illness, or inspiration, we celebrate everyone everywhere who is looking for, and has found, healing and comfort in our soups.

We also want to dedicate this book to our husbands and our children, who motivate and inspire us each day to do all that we can to continue keeping up with them!

Contents

PART III
THE RECIPES

Foreword

I don't know anyone who doesn't want to eat better, feel better, sleep better, and have more energy. We all want to be at our physical, mental, and spiritual best every day, even though we know many of our long-term habits throw up roadblocks that inhibit both our will and our ability to maintain optimal health.

Like you, I've read many books on diet, health, and fitness; like you, I've seen scores of articles bemoaning the rise of obesity, diabetes, stress, and all of the attendant health threats these trends represent. Unfortunately, the complexity of our homeostatic systems—the internal food consumption and regulation signals our bodies send to our brains—makes it difficult for many people to maintain a healthy weight. To make things worse, we often fail to incorporate enough of the right foods that maximize the process of heat production in the body, which can enhance energy levels and metabolism by supporting more efficient calorie burning and lower fat stores.

It is important at every age to find balance among body, mind, and behavior to reduce the burden of chronic ailments and benefit holistic health. And as with so many things in life, prevention is indeed nine-tenths of the cure. Since 2010, I have been working with my colleagues at Massachusetts General Hospital and Harvard Medical School to further the field of integrative medicine research, specifically in adolescents with anxiety and stress conditions. In my private practice, I use functional medicine treatments to address a host of other common and chronic medical complaints. What we often discover is that a series of small adjustments can support long-term change and a healthier overall lifestyle.

Souping is one such adjustment. One of the things I love about this book is its focus on balance; "soup" is no mere four-letter word. Vivienne and Angela offer tips that are meant to be prescriptive rather than prohibitive, although certainly all of the usual culprits behind unhealthy habits are discouraged—alcohol, processed foods, refined sugars, GMOs (genetically modified organisms), and the like. It's helpful to think of the foods and strategies here as evolutionary rather than revolutionary. There's nothing in this book designed to shock your system or starve you into your clothes, neither of which promotes healthy eating habits.

I often remind my patients that no one is perfect, and this book is not about perfection; it's about balance and common sense, about boosting our body's own healing and restorative systems, about supporting health at the cellular level. It's about incorporating more of the best protein, fiber, and whole foods into our diets for maximum nutrient absorption.

If you're asking yourself what all of this means from a practical standpoint, think of souping as an easy and cost-effective way to combat inflammation, heart disease, weight gain, fatigue, and joint pain while promoting glowing skin and hair, improved memory, reduced stress, organ regeneration, and more natural energy. Incorporating these delicious and easy-to-prepare foods into your diet is a meaningful first step toward improving both intermittent and chronic health conditions. Real food. Real nutrition. Real health. Enjoy!

Nada Milosavljevic, MD, JD,
director, Integrative Health Program,
Massachusetts General Hospital;
instructor, Harvard Medical School,
Boston, Massachusetts, May 2015

Health in a Bottle

We didn't start our soup company, Soupure, with the sole intention of offering a better way to cleanse. In fact, we don't believe our bodies are inherently toxic or that a reasonably healthy person needs to be forced to flush their arteries and intestines of some horrible buildup of plaque or sludge. We wanted to, quite simply, offer a better soup and healthier way of eating. We both loved soup—it could be healing, satisfying, warming, cooling, sweet, savory, and, best of all, completely portable. But we were fed up with trying to find one from the grocery store or a restaurant that wasn't packed with salt, sugar, cream, fillers, preservatives, and other funky stuff. Or, if we did manage to find one that wasn't mucked up with additives, it tasted like ground-up and watered-down vegetables. And while we love our veggies, not even the most hard-core herbivore wants to eat a bowlful of sad, unseasoned, unloved plants or, worst of all, a bowl of what tastes like dirty hot water.

Oddly enough, we'd both reached the conclusion that we were dissatisfied with the current state of our quick-and-easy meal options at the same time—and felt strongly enough to do something about it. Angela was working in private equity at the time, Vivienne in law. We'd met almost fifteen years before when our oldest children went to the same nursery school, and we'd kept in touch ever since—a lunch here, a play date there. It was at one of those get-togethers (coincidentally, over a disappointing bowl of soup) that we discovered we value the same tenets of health: moderation, being in touch with your own body, and not making anything strictly taboo. We lamented the challenge it had become to get tasty, nutritious soups, and marveled at why no one was offering them. We both believed in the healing power of nutrient-rich superfoods, particularly bone broths, and felt it more necessary than ever to give those foods to our bodies. And we wanted to give our kids the tools to make good choices too.

Six months later, we'd both left the security of our jobs to create "health in a bottle," as Vivienne likes to say, otherwise known as truly delicious, non-dairy, non-GMO (genetically modified organism—see "What About GMOs?" on page 49 for why we think this is important), preservative-free, 100 percent good-for-you, whole food–based soups, with no bad stuff added. We wanted to offer options that were sweet and savory, chilled and hot. They could be used to cleanse (for one day, three days, or five), or as supplements in people's everyday diets, whether as a post-workout tonic or a better option for lunch or dinner. Above all, we wanted to make a nourishing, healthful, superior, easily transportable product that our families, friends, and—hopefully—just about everyone else could enjoy.

One of the biggest reasons we created Soupure was because we've always had the nagging suspicion that our food plays a big part in our health—both in alleviating certain conditions and in causing them. Vivienne's father was an identical twin, and he got cancer, but his twin didn't, thus suggesting the lack of a genetic predisposition. It led her to wonder if there's something about our environment and how it affects the body that played a role. Also, as middle-aged women, we couldn't believe how many of our peers felt it was too late to feel their best after being married with children and inactive for some years. It wasn't just that they felt they looked tired or overweight or generally zapped of life, it was that they had mentally submitted to aging and believed it was normal to be out of shape after forty. They'd say things like, "Back in my day…" But it's still your day! Flooding your body with nutrients, minerals, vitamins, and phytochemicals is the foundation for staying resilient, well into your twilight years.

In order to figure out how we could help as many people as possible with our soups, we spoke with Whimsy Anderson, ND, a licensed naturopathic doctor practicing holistic medicine in Los Angeles. We asked her to describe the top complaints, ailments, illnesses, and general low-health indicators that she came across in her office. We can't say we were completely surprised by the results—it was the same collection of grievances that we'd hear time after time among friends and family, or in the general public: digestive disorders, joint pain or arthritis, excess weight, poor immune function, fatigue, heart disease, hormone imbalance, diabetes, and other chronic conditions. If you've so much as glimpsed at the news or watched shows like *The Dr. Oz Show* or *The Doctors*, you know that our collective health has taken a nosedive. Recently, the *Wall Street Journal* reported that roughly two-thirds of American adults—155 million people—are overweight or obese. About half of them have at least one preventable disease, including cardiovascular disease or Type 2 diabetes. The primary culprits? Poor eating habits and physical inactivity.

So we took that list from Dr. Anderson, and we made it our mission statement. We set out to create healing soups and an eating regimen that would provide the body everything it needs, particularly the minerals and nutrients that most people don't have in their daily diets. We started looking at how different whole food ingredients can cure, revive, and regenerate, and those ingredients became our new grocery list (which we'll pass on to you). We wanted the recipes to be as unfussy and simple as possible, so we took our findings to a few chefs to see if we could find a culinary vision that matched ours. We found our super-duo in Joli Robinson and Kelsey De Gracia.

They combined their personal passions for holistic healing with food-based medicine to help us realize our dream. Then we ran our potions by a nutritionist—the brilliant and wise Marlyn Diaz, CN—to make sure they were nutritionally sound, then we tweaked, added, nixed, and mixed. It was a collaborative effort not just to provide a product that was superior to anything we'd seen on the market, but also to create something that we were confident could change people's lives. We called on their expertise again when writing this book, so that we could support our passion for these soups and soup cleansing with their nutritional and wellness know-how.

After we launched Soupure, something magical happened: People started feeling better. Our in-boxes and voice mail were flooded with messages from clients telling us about how their skin conditions had vanished, their chronic symptoms abated, they were losing weight, decreasing their medication, looking better, had more energy, and, best of all, they were *happier*. They felt less bloated, had more regular bowel movements (no such thing as oversharing!), their tummy bulge was gone, and they were more clear-minded. Those who had digestive issues all their lives said their symptoms vanished. Others who were on medication for cancer treatments and could barely keep any food down said they finally felt nourished and satisfied. Our friend Lisa said that she stopped getting muscle spasms in the middle of the night and could finally get sound and restful sleep. But it was when Angela's friend Mara said her yoga instructor asked what she was doing differently because her skin was glowing—and the only answer was having our products on a regular basis—that we knew we were definitely on to something.

One of the questions we've heard most since creating Soupure is, "Why not juice?" Before we started our business, we considered the trend of pressed juice cleanses and the claims around them: the removal of toxins, the promotion of healing, rebuilding and rejuvenation, the possibility of finally fitting into those skinny jeans. We know that people love their fresh-pressed juice. And we get it—those bright, colorful bottles promising a world of goodness and beyond sometimes sound too good to pass up. We both drink pressed juice and find it satisfying as an occasional beverage. Our own personal disappointment, however, came when consuming pressed juices as a cleanse/meal substitute. We just didn't feel our best when consuming many of the options on the market today. We felt jittery, unsettled, irritable, and lacking in energy—classic signs of a sugar overdose! And then there was the starvation. We were actually paying to be *hungry*. We saw our friends also totally upended by their cleanses for the same reasons. They had to stop exercising and sometimes even call in sick to work because it was too difficult to get out of the house. We understand the importance of eating vegetables and fruits daily, but too much juice without the fiber just isn't good for anyone (which we'll talk much more about). Fiber is essential to assisting our bodies in naturally cleansing out all the bad stuff, so why are people trying so hard to eliminate it? And we like the beneficial bacteria and enzymes in our digestive systems, thank you very much—we don't want them flushed out! Above all, we don't think people should have to feel bad to feel great. It's one of the reasons we created this slogan for our cleanse label: "Turns out suffering isn't an ingredient, so we didn't include it." Plus, we couldn't figure out why we'd just throw away one of the best parts of the plant— the fiber! We'll talk much more about the health benefits of keeping some roughage in your diet, but suffice it to say that whole plants were built that way for a reason.

Often people are searching for one specific way to eat—raw, vegan, Paleo, and so on—and it's usually whatever's trendy. That seems to be why the whole cleansing movement started in the first place. We think the best way to "cleanse" is to stop eating and drinking processed and refined foods and start eating more nutrient-dense whole foods. What we discovered in creating our soups is that healthy eating doesn't fit into a tiny box. Food isn't totally "good" or completely "bad." Animal foods can be just as healing as vegetables. Fruit isn't the devil, and neither is (natural) sugar. Some plants are more nutritious when cooked, and others when raw. Fat is your friend! This new wisdom made us question everything that we thought we knew about food, dieting, and cleansing. By surrounding ourselves with smart, informed, and enlightened experts on nutrition and healthful eating, we were able to shift our mind-set from one of strictly counting calories, restricting certain foods (cooked, carbs, fat, animal protein, etc.), and everything else included in the capital "D" Dieting, to understanding that if we fed and nourished our bodies with "clean," high-fiber, whole foods, we could create the most effective cleansing system in the universe! It made us realize that maybe we had found a new "cleansing" trend: *balance.*

Sound Familiar?

According to Whimsy Anderson, ND, these are the most common concerns her patients want resolved, and what we set out to address with our soups (in no particular order):

1. **"Los Angeles syndrome":** A series of conditions resulting from hectic urban life. Whether or not you're in L.A., we think you'll find this syndrome all too relatable, because it's plaguing U.S. cities nationwide. This urban malaise usually includes symptoms of **anxiety, depression, panic attacks, sleep disorders**, and **extreme fatigue**.
2. **Hormone imbalance or hormone replacement options:** In demand from women in their early forties to late sixties, as well as those trying to get pregnant or recovering post-partum.
3. **Weight loss:** Individuals struggling to maintain an ideal body weight and looking to find a solution that's lifelong and sustainable.
4. **Digestive disorders:** A common complaint that can include **nausea and vomiting** (due to **morning sickness** or **influenza**),

dysbiosis (poor digestion due to overgrowth of toxic forms of bacteria in the gastrointestinal system), **acid reflux**, and **pancreatic insufficiency**.

5. **Arthritis and joint pain:** Often seen in patients over forty but also found in young athletes.

6. **Immune support:** Everything from warding off the common cold to concerns about general immune health and cancer risk.

7. **Libido enhancement and growth hormone support:** For men who are looking to improve their potency and gain muscle safely.

8. **Antiaging:** For the very large number of people in search of tonics or remedies that will delay the aging process and lead to a younger, fresher appearance.

9. **Inflammation and autoimmune diseases:** Including conditions such as lupus, rheumatoid arthritis, multiple sclerosis, inflammatory bowel disease (IBD), Type 1 diabetes, and psoriasis.

10. **Coronary heart disease:** Whether these individuals have already had a heart attack or are looking to prevent one, and addressing issues such as **high blood pressure** and **high cholesterol**.

11. **Cancer:** Whether it's seeking **preventive measures, alternative remedies**, or **adjunct therapy** in addition to conventional treatments.

12. **Type 2 diabetes and metabolic syndrome:** Epidemic conditions that are often the result of **obesity**.

13. **Detoxification:** The desire to clean out the liver, kidney, and gastrointestinal tract in order to reap many health benefits, including addressing most, if not all, of the concerns on this list.

Okay, so we're not claiming to hold the key to universal truths—we make soup, people!—but we do believe that a clean and balanced diet goes a long way toward curing your health conditions, from the nagging to the serious and chronic. We're willing to bet that if you're reading this book, you're not feeling as great as you'd like. And that you're also tired of being told that you need to suffer in order to lose weight or to feel good again, whether it's battling through hunger and deprivation or giving up foods that taste good and bring you joy. But we believe that if you're sick or tired or burned out, then you've already suffered enough. Learning how to nourish your body is all about giving, not taking away. It's *giving* your cells, organs, blood, and tissues every nutrient they need to be in their happy place. It's *giving* yourself food that satisfies, inspires, and just plain tastes good. And it's *giving* yourself the life and body that you've always wanted. The bottom line is that a balanced, high-fiber diet made up of whole fresh foods is nature's best cleansing and detoxing system. It increases the speed and efficiency of the digestive system and helps your organs rid your body of internal and environmental toxins. Why spend your money on expensive weight-loss supplements, pills, or fancy systems when you can spend it in the produce department and give your body what it really needs to cleanse and work at its optimal levels?

But why would we just give away some of the most popular recipes from Soupure? Because when you're happy, healthy, and vibrant, it makes a happier, healthier, more vibrant world for all of us. Knowing that these soups are amazingly curative, we want to offer them in a way that can create long-lasting health for anyone. Young and old, our soups are for everyone. And we couldn't be more excited to share them with you.

PEACE, LOVE, AND SOUP

Vivienne's Story

When I was in high school and college, I struggled with an eating disorder. Even after I got better, though, I still had trouble kicking an "it's all or nothing" attitude when it came to food. I've always been searching for a way of eating that offered a little balance and a little forgiveness.

Meanwhile, I was leading an incredibly busy life. I was working at a big law firm and then at a studio as an entertainment lawyer with three kids and a dad with cancer. I didn't have time to make myself the kind of food I knew I should be eating. And, if you don't have time to cook a healthy meal and you want something quick and delicious, you're going to reach for a bag of chips. You can't just grab a head of broccoli or a bunch of kale and eat it. Well, you could, but it wouldn't taste very good. I didn't want my daughter to make the same mistakes that I made. So that meant providing food choices that are not only healthful but also convenient, and, more important, balanced. I wanted my daughter—and my sons—to see firsthand that eating well doesn't mean too little of one thing and too much of another. Deprivation is not health. Nor is eating an endless surplus of leafy greens and miso broth. To me, health is creating a foundation of life-giving foods—and then not beating yourself up if you have that slice of cake, or a cookie, or a burger.

During that time, I saw how many people were buying fresh-pressed juice and using it to cleanse, so I figured that that many people couldn't be wrong. I did several pressed juice cleanses—whenever I wanted to lose a little weight or detox—but I didn't look forward to it. I usually do some form of exercise (whether it's a hike, yoga, spin class, or run with the dogs) every day, and I didn't want to do anything, not even walk, while on a juice cleanse. I had a headache, I was lethargic and jittery thanks to the rush of sugar from the defibered fruits and vegetables, and I wasn't satisfied. While I did lose weight, I felt like it was through starvation, and that was a tough price to pay for the "prize." (Not only that, but I gained back all the weight when I returned to my regular eating habits and sometimes even gained more weight!) I wished that I could do all the things I read about with a juice cleanse—flush out the toxins, give my body a break from digesting food so that it could repair and heal, bring down any puffiness or bloating—but with "real" whole food in whatever form it is most nutritiously consumed.

That's when I started thinking about soup. I was always order-ing soup in restaurants; it was soothing and satisfying and filling. But my only soup choices for everyday meals were oversalted take-out or underseasoned, watery "healthy" options. Then one day I was walking down the street and passed a juice shop with a line out the door. That's when the lightbulb went on. *What if I started a business that sold whole food–based soups (both hot and cold) that were delicious and nutritious? I wondered. And what if they were completely portable? Packaging them in glass bottles instead of cups or bowls so people would consider soup the same way they'd been turning to juice? What if soups could be combined in a way to assist the digestive system in naturally cleansing and restoring itself?*

At lunch one day with my friend Angela, I brought up this idea and, lo and behold, I wasn't the only one looking for this kind of solution. After Angela and I launched Soupure, we could barely keep up with demand. The only downside of turning our passion for soup into a business is that it's selling out! So I can't always get all the soup I want. But when I do have it in my life and use it for cleansing—even if it's just for one day—I feel so much better. I have more energy, my tummy's a little flatter, and my mind is clearer. Normally I need a supplement for irritable bowel syndrome, but I don't need it when I'm eating the soups. Most important, though, it's made me more aware of what I should be eating to feel my best, and it helps my family learn the same lessons.

Angela's Story

I've always loved soup, and I've always made tons of it at home, whether it be chicken soups or vegetable purees. But leaving an extremely lucrative career in investment finance to start a soup company—that was certainly not something I thought would happen.

Even though I've always been a seeker when it comes to finding something healthy to eat, I all but starved myself in high school and college, so as an adult I really wanted to find balanced eating habits that supported how I liked to look but still made me feel nourished. With this goal in mind, my journey to Soupure began. But truth be told, it really started with my kids.

First, my son, Hudson, had the flu, so I got him some chicken soup from a Jewish deli. I realized after the soup had sat in the fridge overnight that it hadn't congealed—a telltale sign that the broth hadn't been made with the bones. So I called a few delis, and sure enough, no one was making it with the bones. But that's what makes it Jewish penicillin! There's no way to get all the biotin, collagen, and nutrients if you're not simmering the chicken bones for at least three to four hours.

The next thing that happened was my daughter Jacqlyn really wanted to find a healthy, non-dairy tomato basil soup. I didn't have a great recipe, so I went to the supermarket to see what options were out there. I found it almost impossible to find a version that didn't have any additives or preservatives. Even the companies touting their products as organic, whole-heart, whole earth, and so on usually had cream as the second or third ingredient. I finally found one at a restaurant that specialized in clean food, but their soup tasted like a can of tomato paste. I knew that there had to be a way to make it better. There is no reason why a soup needs to have cream to be delicious. And let's face it, those of us choosing vegetable soups at restaurants are trying to be healthy, so do we really want the cream? If I am having cream, then I am having lobster bisque.

The third thing to happen was my kids, led by my daughter Sabrina, dragged me to a juice place, and I ordered a citrus juice. I'd had only about four ounces of it when I started perspiring on my upper lip and felt jittery. It was a clear sign that my body, which gets very little sugar from my normal diet, was on overload. I did a little research when I got home and found that some pressed juices can have as much as *39 grams of unbound sugar in one little bottle.* That's almost as much as a bagful of chocolate chip cookies! Cap'n Crunch, look out, you have got competition. Okay, so I'm not going to equate juiced greens and apples to processed cereals and treats, but it really made me think. What if there was a better way to get all of these nutrients, and why does eating healthy and watching your weight need to be so difficult?

I realized that I could combine the portable, five-servings-of-veggies-in-a-bottle, instant-gratification appeal and time-tested power of soup and meet a very clear need not just in the market, but also in my own fridge. So when Vivienne and I realized we shared the same vision, it was a no-brainer.

Since incorporating these soups into my life I feel cleaner, healthier, and even more energetic (hard to believe since people usually call me the Energizer Bunny, but yes, even more energy). Whereas I normally would fall into a rut of eating the same foods every day or week, the soups help me stuff as many as a hundred different nutrients into just one day with a variety of fruits, vegetables, legumes, seeds, nuts, spices, and herbs. My kids love the soups too. Even when they complain about eating breakfast before going to school, I know if I get them to suck down a delicious smoothie, they'll get something healthy in their bodies (that also happens to be great brain food and helps them focus and perform in school and in sports). And instead of Gatorade, which it seems like they're always drinking at sports practice, now they can have an Energize, which is a strawberry cashew smoothie that has tons of vitamins and minerals, plus no preservatives, no dyes, and nothing artificial—but all they know is that it tastes like a delicious smoothie and they love it! It's been a great way of giving my family healthier choices, and an amazing insurance policy for getting nourishing food when life happens. I never thought I would leave private equity, but finding better nutrition and healthy fast-food alternatives for my on-the-go kids and myself became a priority. Saving them from the traps of crazy diets to lose weight and finding a better way to help their bodies recover from sports was a must. Now, with Soupure and with this book, I want to share our soups with everyone to help them feel better, healthier, and happier.

Part I

THE GOOD,
THE BAD, AND
THE SOLUTION

1

Getting Healthy in a
Toxic World

We know you're pretty excited to dive headfirst into our program and all things soup—we would be too!—but first it's important to understand why whole food–based cleansing is so essential, and why adding these soups to your diet will be so life-changing.

To get to the bottom of what's so healthy, let's talk about what's *not*: chemicals, pesticides, synthetic hormones, additives, fillers, fake vitamins, fake nutrients, fake food, and toxins, toxins, toxins. Basically, everything you've most likely been putting in your body up until now.

We can't blame you; most Americans have been duped into eating a diet filled with "food" that's crammed with ingredients they can barely pronounce and loaded with salt and refined sugar. Food manufacturers spend a ton of money trying to convince us that if we just buy this box of X or bottle of Y, we'll have all the vitamins and nutrients we need with fewer calories! Less fat! More fiber! Do you really believe it?

The truth is, if our ancestors came back today and stood in the middle of a grocery store, they most likely wouldn't recognize any of the items on offer. Humans didn't start out on this planet with big food factories, right? We were picking berries and nuts, killing animals, fishing, and growing our own food. As we like to think of it: If it didn't have a mother or wasn't grown from the earth, then it's usually not natural or healthy. So essentially much of our food is no longer food. This is so much the case that the need for "organic" foods was born. No one thought about organic food when there were no food factories and we were not polluting our land and food. Now we are using pesticides, chemicals, and hormones to grow our fruits, vegetables, and animals bigger more quickly.

These faux-food elements are wreaking havoc on our bodies. They are taking a toll on our digestive systems, immune systems, respiratory systems, even our brains! It's no wonder that obesity is out of control, allergies and autoimmune diseases are on the rise, and conditions such as chronic fatigue syndrome, fibromyalgia, multiple sclerosis, Alzheimer's disease, heart disease, and cancer are becoming more pervasive. The food that we're being told to put in our mouths is so far from what nature intended that we have created toxic pollutants in ourselves, and they are making us fat, sick, old, and tired. And to add insult to injury, we add more toxins to our bodies through the (unfiltered) water we drink, the air we breathe, and the way we live (yes, stress is a toxin!).

We're already inflicting damage on our bodies just by living—we're aging every day!—expending tons of energy bringing in oxygen and moving around, tending to our daily tasks. This means our bodies are constantly working on repairs; we're always a little behind when it comes to healing and replenishing. But if we're not supporting the body and are instead breaking it down, then we start to see illness, chronic conditions, energy depletion, and so on.

But we wouldn't bum you out with all this if we didn't have a special secret to share: You can change all that! You can clean up and help your body naturally detoxify. You can restore all your systems by giving them the nutrients they need to heal, rebuild, and revitalize. You can give your body an improved ability to fight off disease, reduce inflammation, and slow the aging process. Once you learn how to regularly clear out your body with our cleanse, we promise that you will look better *and* feel better. You'll lose weight, have more energy, and feel vibrant, sexy, and alive. We promise!

For the past five years I've suffered from an autoimmune illness (AI) that results in chronic sinusitis, daily sinus headaches, massive fatigue, and brain fog. I've struggled every day, feeling like I have a bad cold or flu. I've had two surgeries, been prescribed thirty-seven types of medication, and been treated by nine specialists. The doctors could only get me about 30 percent better. That's when I began treating my AI with diet alone, and I'm feeling 80 percent better. I've found that Soupure's unique clean ingredients greatly decrease inflammation in my body and digestive system. These soups are also helping improve gut health, as well as my adrenal fatigue.

On my third day of cleansing, I felt so good I had to sit down and think about the last time I felt that healthy. It was five years ago, before I got sick. The weight loss is just an added bonus. I wish I figured this out years ago, but I'm finally on my way to better health and, most important, feeling good every day!

—Caitlyn M.

TOXINS 101

It seems like these days everyone is throwing around the word "toxic" to describe just about everything we come into contact with.

Is this Chicken Little syndrome, or is the world really that toxic? And what the heck is a toxin, anyway?

A toxin is a substance that, simply put, damages the body. And unfortunately, they really do pop up pretty much anywhere you look. There are toxins that we make (pesticides and other industrial chemicals), toxins in our water (chlorine, heavy metals like lead and mercury, and even traces of pharmaceutical medications), toxins in our air (mold and mildew, fumes, smoke), toxins in our food (additives, fillers, stabilizers, and synthetic coloring and flavoring), and even toxins in our beauty and health products, cleaning products, furniture, and clothes. In fact, we're living among over eighty-five thousand chemicals. While many of these have been tested for their toxicity threshold in the human body (for instance, a small amount of mercury or lead is technically "okay"), there's no way to know what that magic number really is, how much you're really being exposed to, or what's happening when all these substances interact with one another. All these toxins can build up in your body and cause all kinds of harm to your cells and tissues, resulting in discomfort, disease, or chronic conditions. It's called "toxic burden."[1]

The good news is that your body has a built-in detoxification system made up of your cells, blood, skin, and a number of organs (like your liver and kidneys, which we'll talk about in more detail in a bit). They work hard day in and day out to keep these toxins from permanently taking up residence. Problem is, it's a system that worked best a hundred years ago when the air and water were cleaner and things like ethoxylated surfactants weren't in our face cleansers or butylated hydroxytoluene in our breakfast cereal. Now, though, that system is, for most of us, struggling to keep up with our modern food supply, industrial pollutants, and all the other insults we expose it to on a daily basis. Our detoxification systems are overwhelmed by our toxic burden, and as a result we're seeing illness, fatigue, headaches, mood disorders, and all those nagging aches and pains that aren't contributing to a healthy, happy life.

What Does Toxic Load Look Like?

When the body fills with toxins, you start to see damage at the cellular level. This is what that could look like to you:

Accelerated aging

Achy joints

Disease, such as diabetes, cancer, high blood pressure

Dry hair and brittle nails

Dry mouth and bad breath

Fatigue

Headaches

Infection

Memory loss or "brain fog"

Mood disorders, such as anxiety, depression, mood swings

Pain

Poor sleep

Skin issues, such as eczema, dull skin, acne, rashes

Sore muscles

Weight gain

Toxins affect our health on a cellular level. Two of the main ways they inflict damage are *oxidative stress* and *inflammation*.

OXIDATIVE STRESS

In a nutshell: Our tissues and cells are always rusting. Just like a shovel or toy wagon left out in the rain and mottled by damaging oxidization, our cells too are constantly battling being overtaken by harmful agents in the body.

It looks a little something like this: The cells in our active organs (think muscles, heart, brain) have little energy factories called mitochondria. These mechanisms turn the food we eat and oxygen we breathe into energy. This fuel, which runs the body, is called adenosine triphosphate, or ATP. But even though this is a highly beneficial function of the body, it also creates dangerous by-products. These include highly toxic free radicals. Not to get too textbook on you, but free radicals are essentially rogue, unstable atoms that are looking to snatch electrons from other molecules in the body in order to make themselves whole or stable again. In doing so, they create even more unstable molecules, which then go on the hunt for their missing electrons. It creates a chain reaction that causes extensive damage throughout the body. This is compounded by the already burdensome toxic load the body carries, since toxins coming in from the outside (anything we're eating, breathing, drinking, exposed to, or rubbing on our skin) can also create oxidization. The result is—you guessed it—disease.

Luckily, the body isn't defenseless to these attacks. It protects itself by creating a physical barrier that can contain the marauding free radicals. Its shield? Antioxidants. That's right, those mysterious entities that people are always celebrating in their blueberries and face creams. It turns out there's really something to them.

Antioxidants come from the food you eat (the good stuff, that is). Plants—primarily fruits and vegetables—contribute vitamins A, C, and E; coenzyme Q10; manganese; iodine; and polyphenols, which lock down free radicals and neutralize them. They also help to heal and repair the mitochondria.

Without a diet rich in plants, though, your body can't produce enough antioxidants to protect itself from oxidation. That's why we've loaded our soups with fruits, vegetables, nuts, and other ingredients packed with antioxidants, so that during your cleanse and long afterward you can give your body the strong defense it needs. And because the soups are so much easier on your digestion than your regular diet thanks to how they're cooked and blended (more on this in a bit), your body is expending less cellular energy. When that happens, free radical production drops.

INFLAMMATION

The other way that toxins can damage cells is through inflammation. "Inflammation," much like "toxins" and "antioxidants," has become a sort of buzzword recently. But it too has a very justified place in our health vocabulary.

The easiest way to wrap your head around inflammation is to think about what happens when you bang your hand and it turns black and blue. It's inflamed. Or think about eczema or acne—that's inflammation on the outside (which is usually a result of something happening on the inside). Sometimes our bodies' inflammatory response can be a positive thing. It's a process our immune systems use to fight off bacteria, viruses, and other pathogens that could cause harm. It's also inflammatory when white blood cells go in to support healing. But while inflammation is a powerful and beneficial short-term response to fight infection, it's very harmful when it becomes chronic. That's when you start seeing damage to the body that manifests like puffiness, stuffiness, bloat, skin eruptions, headaches, cholesterol imbalance, blood challenges, chronic pain, diseases such as heart disease and arthritis, and brain-related conditions such as Parkinson's and Alzheimer's disease.

Toxins, whether from our insides or the outside, can trigger the inflammatory response. And when the response is set off by toxins, it's typically more intense than if it were simply responding to an injury SOS. What happens is the immune system starts misreading our own tissues as foreign invaders, leading to an autoimmune response—or the body attacking itself. This is the culprit behind many food-related allergies, as well as diseases such as lupus, multiple sclerosis, and scleroderma.[2] The more prevalent inflammation becomes in the body, the greater free radical production there is. The more free radical production there is, the more oxidation occurs. And the more oxidation occurs, the more inflammation results, because the body is trying to keep up with fixing all that damage.[3] Essentially, our toxic burden is creating a constant loop of damage in our bodies.

Inflammation is kind of like an iceberg in the ocean—often we see just the tip, but what really is going on is much deeper and pervasive, and often the cause of health challenges and diseases. It can be difficult to pinpoint where inflammation is stemming from, but food can be a huge source of the problem. When you remove foods that are known to cause inflammation—dairy, gluten, corn, and soy, just to name a few—and add foods that quell unnecessary inflammation, you can start to create shifts in the body. Your skin might also clear up, you'll lose weight, the stuffiness and puffiness will diminish, the bloat will go down, and your body will return to a more balanced state.

THE TOP SIX INFLAMMATORY FOODS

We recommend steering clear of these foods, which is why we don't include them in our soups or in our recipes:

Gluten. Gluten is a protein found in wheat and related grains like rye. In breads, it is the "glue" that holds them together. While gluten is not intrinsically bad for you, it's more a function of how our wheat is grown. Here in the United States, most strains of wheat are hard for the body to digest,[4] compounded by the fact that they're genetically modified (see "What About GMOs?" on page 49, but suffice it to say that genetically modified organisms are wreaking havoc on you and on the planet).[5] Plus, when you strip out all the nutrients of wheat to create white flour, you're creating a product that's even more taxing on the body's systems. Many people confuse "gluten" with "starch," since these terms are often used to describe things like pasta and bread. However, some starch is excellent for the body, whereas gluten—sometimes not so much. Starch is the carbohydrate component found in most foods. Rice, for example, is a gluten-free food but is a starch. So too are potatoes, lentils, and quinoa, just to name a few. We believe that including starchy foods in the diet is a good thing, though in moderation.

Dairy. The casein from cow's milk is hard for many people's systems to break down and for most people is inflammatory.[6] It also doesn't help that many animals are raised with hormones and antibiotics, which compound the inflammatory effect on our bodies. Raw dairy is a different story, and some people can tolerate it.

Corn. It's a moldy crop containing mycotoxins (the toxic metabolic by-products of fungi),[7] and is often GMO (see "What About GMOs?" on page 49). That said, incorporating a small amount of fresh organic corn into your diet can be beneficial for some.

Processed soy. The challenge with soy is that much of it has been highly processed (think "isolated soy," which you will find on the label of most processed foods). Another problem is that almost all non-organic soy crops in the United States have been genetically modified, which we'll talk more about in a bit. But the primary concern is that these crops are often sprayed with herbicides like Roundup, which contains glyphosate, classified as "probably carcinogenic" by the World Health Organization.[8]

Soy in all its forms can contribute to a host of health challenges. It contains phytic acid, a toxic compound that is challenging for the body to digest. It can inhibit the body from absorbing iron, calcium, zinc, and magnesium. Soy also has protease inhibitors, which can block some of the enzymes the body needs in order to digest protein.[9] Then there's the phytoestrogen issue. Research has shown that the estrogen in soy can act as an endocrine disruptor, which can interfere with your body's hormonal function and lead to things like cancer.[10] And additionally consider that soy is what they feed to pigs and cows to make them fat. Think about that anytime you reach for ice cream, yogurt, chips, or any processed product that warns "made with soy."

That said, unprocessed and fermented soy made from non-GMO (see "What About GMOs?" on page 49) soybeans is a traditionally healing food (think tempeh and miso). Asian countries are known to eat soy for its health benefits, though they consume it in much smaller amounts than we do in America. These products can be tolerated well by some, and for these reasons we include them in small amounts in some of our soups (more on this later).

Refined and processed sugars. These sweeteners have been stripped of any kind of nutrition, and they deplete the body, as well as trigger and accelerate the aging process. Sugar—and its other forms like high-fructose corn syrup, cane sugar, evaporated cane juice (organic and otherwise), beet sugar, palm sugar, malt syrup, and pretty much any ingredient you see ending in "-ose"—causes inflammation, leads to weight gain and diabetes, and is linked to cancer.[11] Not to mention that it makes you feel really crummy. Artificial sweeteners such as aspartame, saccharin, and sucralose (otherwise known as NutraSweet, Equal, Sweet'N Low, and Splenda) are lab-made by-products from things like coal tar and antiulcer drugs. While there is conflicting research about the long-term effects of fake sweeteners on humans,[12] common sense tells us that they're not doing you or your health any favors. Don't worry; we won't take all your sweet treats away. Natural sweeteners such as dates, dried apricots, coconut sugar, raw honey, coconut, and maple syrup can actually benefit the body while still satisfying your sweet tooth.

MSG. Otherwise known as monosodium glutamate, MSG is one of the food industry's favorite ingredients because of its delicious salty, umami flavor that you can achieve with a fraction of the cooking effort—especially in soups. As neighborhood butcher shops become a thing of the past, fewer people are using bones and other animal bits to get deep, rich flavor naturally (which is how our ancestors used to do it). Now we've been promised that same result with a little packet of powder. Unfortunately, MSG is a neurotoxin that disrupts the nervous system.[13] It lurks in processed food and is sometimes hidden behind names like "natural flavor," "autolyzed yeast," and "hydrolyzed protein." Any packaged product that comes with a flavor packet most likely contains MSG.

Inflammation and Acidity

One of the major causes of inflammation in the body is too much acidity in the system. Ideally, your body would rest at a perfect pH level between 7.365 and 7.4. That means that it's not too acidic, and also not too alkaline (though it leans in that direction). The body is constantly looking to maintain that balance so it and all your vital organs can function at their peak ability. When you ingest foods and liquids, the end products (after digestion and assimilation) result in an acid ash, alkaline-acid ash, or alkaline ash. Plants and vegetables are known to have an alkaline ash, while white flour and sugar have an acid ash. Each has an alkaline- or acid-forming effect on the body. One of the ways the body brings itself into balance is through its own buffering system. Eating a highly acid-forming diet over time can disrupt some of the buffering or balancing effects of the body. So what you eat largely informs your body's pH balance, though it's also affected by factors such as stress, toxins, cigarettes, and drugs.

If your diet is high in pro-inflammatory foods like white flour, refined sugar, meat, cheese, and processed food (which create excess acid waste), then there's a good chance that your body is too acidic. Research shows that a more acidic body is more prone to disease.[14] You might see symptoms such as frequent flus and colds; digestive issues such as heartburn, acid reflux, or irritable bowel syndrome; allergies; acne or eczema; joint pain; asthma; hormonal imbalance (especially less-forgiving PMS); depression or anxiety; low energy; low libido; migraines or headaches; and even Crohn's disease, multiple sclerosis, and cancer. What's happening is that your body is using its precious energy to rebalance its pH levels and return to homeostasis instead of on nourishing and repairing the body.

On the other end of the spectrum are healing, alkaline (low-inflammatory) foods, which support the body in its overall health by helping it stay in balance. These primarily include fresh, plant-based foods, especially fruits and vegetables, and are the foundation of our soups.

Our cleanses are formulated so that you can counteract an over-acidic system, primarily through the soups and also through simple daily practices such as drinking infused alkaline waters or plain water with a spritz of lemon juice (which, though acidic outside the body, is alkaline and healing when taken internally), as well as breathing and exercising. These measures aren't just healing, they're also potent preventive medicine.

Before beginning a cleanse, we recommend checking your pH level. Most pharmacies carry strips for a simple urine test, or you can order them online.

Examples of Alkaline Foods

Almonds	Curry
Apples	Figs
Artichokes	Flaxseeds
Arugula	Garlic
Asparagus	Ginger
Avocados	Grapefruits
Bananas	Grapes
Beets	Green beans
Bell peppers	Hemp seeds
Broccoli	Honey
Brussels sprouts	Leeks
Buckwheat groats	Lemons
Cabbage	Lentils
Carrots	Limes
Cauliflower	Melons
Celery	Okra
Chia seeds	Olive oil
Cinnamon	Onions
Coconuts	Oranges
Cucumbers	Parsley

Peaches
Pears
Peas
Pomegranates
Pumpkin
Spirulina
Squash
Radishes
Rutabaga

Sea salt
Sesame seeds
Sprouts
Tomatoes
Turnips
Watercress
Wheatgrass
Zucchini

Also alkaline are non–chemically grown leafy greens such as spinach, kale, collards, Swiss chard, and romaine, as well as seaweeds such as kombu, hijiki, dulse, and wakame.

Acidic (Pro-Inflammatory) Foods

Alcohol
Caffeine
Conventional meat
Corn
Dairy
Gluten

Grains
Processed foods
Refined sugar
Soda
Soy

MEET THE PLAYERS

As you get ready to learn more about our soups and cleanse programs, we think it's important to have a basic understanding of what's going on under the hood—that is, in your own body. Every vitamin, mineral, and nutrient that goes into your body is allocated to an indispensable bodily function. And when it comes to our soups, we paid particular attention to the nutrients required to support the organs and processes that are doing their damnedest to keep your body clean, tidy, and of course healthy.

The Cleanup Crew

As we mentioned earlier, the body has its own detoxification system. You support this well-oiled machine when you limit the number of toxins coming into the body and increase the number of nutrients. It also helps that when you eat blended and cooked soup—which requires very little energy from your digestive system because it's already "predigested," or blended—you're allowing these mechanisms to focus solely on essential maintenance rather than constantly playing catch-up.

The liver. This is the filter of the body. It sieves out bad guys from the blood, including chemicals, heavy metals, unnecessary hormones, and other toxins. It converts these toxins to a water-soluble state so that they can be excreted through the kidneys. It plays a key role in relieving digestive issues, such as sluggish metabolism, gas, bloating, and constipation. It also regulates blood sugar levels, which when out of balance can cause sugar cravings, fatigue, and brain fog. Without a healthy liver, you may suffer from hormonal imbalances that can cause headaches, mood swings, and depression.[15] And a liver overstressed by the consumption of processed and refined foods can lead to inflammatory diseases like diabetes, arthritis, high blood pressure, and autoimmune diseases. So think of the liver as you would the oil filter on your car—it gets pretty nasty when it gets backed up with pollutants. We want to love the liver and lighten its load. If you remove chemicals and toxins from your body, it can do its job better. Eating foods that benefit your liver are also essential to keeping this powerhouse functioning optimally.

The kidneys. The kidneys are a powerful chemical factory that removes waste products from the body, helps regulate blood pressure, stimulates red blood cell production, and helps the body maintain adequate calcium levels. In traditional Chinese medicine, the kidneys are considered to be the center of where your chi, or life force, emanates from.

The intestines. The intestines are all about getting the junk out of the trunk. They are crucial for processing the waste that comes from your food and eliminating it from the body, as well as transferring the nutritional value of that food into the cells of your body. They serve as a drainpipe for waste produced as a result of metabolic functions within the body, as well as for toxic substances absorbed through your lungs and skin. Essentially, all the waste of the body comes out through the intestinal tract, so it's important to keep it clean, vibrant, and healthy. Otherwise it can get backed up with all kinds of bad stuff. This is a huge vote for fiber!

The blood. Your blood feeds every cell, tissue, gland, organ, and organ system in your body. It carries nutrients and oxygen throughout the body, making sure these systems stay strong. It also functions as a highway of sorts, so keeping the blood cleansed, pH-balanced, and moving helps sweep unwanted toxins through and out of your body.

The cells. Everything comes back to the cells. They are the fundamental units of life, making up all your tissues and organs. When they are functioning well, they are constantly communicating with one another, responding to your environment and to the signals they receive from your actions. They are responsible for making up the processes that produce energy and heat, remove waste, and regenerate, as well as produce antibodies, hormones, and neurotransmitters. Perhaps most important, they keep your DNA safe from damage. Research has shown that a poor diet—one low in antioxidants and other important phytonutrients—and exposure to toxins can cause your DNA to become damaged.[16] This can cause your cells to die prematurely, leading to compromised tissue or inflammation, and can even trigger certain diseases, especially cancer.

The Wingman

The lymphatic system. This series of tissues and organs' primary objective is to support the circulatory and immune systems. It returns fluid lost in tissues to the blood in order to maintain homeostasis, the balance that is so important to good health. It also serves as a kind of piping system, helping to drain waste from the body, especially potentially harmful bacteria, therefore helping to fight infection and disease. Sometimes, however, if large amounts of toxic material are floating around your body, it can get clogged in the lymph nodes (which are found in the neck, under the arms, and around the groin, among other areas). The lymphatic system doesn't have a pump the way your circulatory system does, so its fluid can get stagnant. Exercise is helpful for moving that waste out, and there are even yoga poses that are specifically designed to help lymphatic drainage (especially inversions).

The Unsung Hero

The gut. The gut has become quite a celebrity lately, and for good reason. We host more life in our bellies than there are stars in the galaxy, and these beneficial bacteria provide a number of essential functions, including aiding digestion and supporting the immune system. That's right—the once lowly gut is intrinsically tied to our ability to stay healthy. Our gut flora—or microbiome, as you may have heard it called—has the ability to identify, attack, and destroy many invading pathogens, as well as produce a number of nutrients and biochemicals that boost our immune systems. In fact, numerous studies have linked the gut microbiome to a range of body functions such as appetite, cravings, mood, and emotion.[17] The gut even appears to help maintain healthy brain function!

Unfortunately, the same factors that have compromised our health over the past few decades are also having an effect on our guts. Eating too many high-inflammatory foods can suppress these little gastrointestinal troops, as can too many prescription medications, especially antibiotics. When we deplete or imbalance our gut flora, it inhibits our ability to absorb all the nutrients we take in. It also can lead to digestive, autoimmune, neurological, and even psychological disorders. Ironically, some cleanses can actually deplete your gut flora because they flush out all the bacteria, good and bad. This is neither necessary nor healthy.

The best way to nourish your gut and enhance and support your gut flora is the same way you nourish the rest of your body: by boosting your intake of nutritious foods (think whole, unprocessed, and unrefined foods) while decreasing your toxin exposure and intake of inflammation-promoting foods. It's also beneficial to eat gut-healing foods such as gelatin and collagen-rich bone broth, as well as probiotic foods. These include kimchi, miso, and pickled foods, which contain live beneficial bacteria.

EATING TO DETOX

To call our program a "cleanse" is almost cheating, because it's really just boosting your own natural detoxification system. Since your body's internal cleansing system *loves* food, especially food that provides care and sustenance for all its functions, we've taken care to include in our soups all the nutrients that help boost kidney, blood, liver, and cell health, as well as those that help heal the gut. Among a whole buffet of others, there's iron-rich leafy greens and legumes to create strong blood and healthy kidneys; essential fatty acids from seeds, healthy oils, and nuts to create more supple cell membranes; sulfur-packed foods like garlic and onions to help your liver rid your body of toxins; and cultured food like miso to restore healthy bacteria like lactobacilli to the digestive tract. By consuming these foods, we cleanse and detox twenty-four hours a day.

2

Finding Your Sexy

What is sexy? To us, it's glowing skin, confidence, energy, vitality, a body that's lean and efficient, a mind that's clear and sharp, and a spirit that's in love with life. These qualities aren't age-dependent, and they're yours for the taking. It simply comes down to what you eat, how you live, and keeping a positive frame of mind.

Nature has used the same rules for vitality for a long time—if you break the rules, your skin doesn't glow, your body and your brain feel sluggish, and chronic ailments start to creep up. Depriving your body of the nourishment it needs from a variety of whole foods can get pretty ugly, inside and out.

That's why we formulated a better, easier way to get all the good stuff—everything you need to look and feel amazing. In addition to all the benefits we talked about in the previous chapter, there are proteins; the smart energy contained in good fats and complex carbohydrates; an array of colorful, powerful, disease-fighting phytonutrients; and loads of fiber, which is crucial for cleaning out all the gunk that's built up over time in your intestinal tract and is slowing you down. These things combined are the key to optimal health, and when you find that balance, that's pretty darn sexy.

Being hypersensitive to everything in my environment (fragrances, foods, etc.) has forced me to become extremely educated about what I put on me, in me, and have around me. I love Soupure, as their soups are made with only the healthiest organic ingredients, which taste amazing and are completely satisfying! Whoever heard of healthy fast food? Now people tell me my skin has a wonderful glow, and then I share my Soupure secret. It's better than any makeup could ever do.

—Morgan R.

DON'T LET CHRONIC SYMPTOMS TAKE YOUR SEXY AWAY

We've listed a lot of symptoms of an unhealthy body, and chances are at least one or two apply to you. So please hear us when we say: Don't let your symptoms dominate you. *You are not your symptoms!* So often, people start to think, *Oh, I'm just a moody person, I just don't sleep well, I am too tired or stressed to exercise,* or *This is just my lot in life because I was born with a slow metabolism.* But the truth is that these are all things we have a lot of control over. And many times it starts with the foods that you put into your body. Too little and you slow your metabolism down and throw your body into starvation mode. Too much and you feel sluggish and lethargic.

We can help you make food and exercise your friends. *There is hope, even if you struggle with chronic symptoms.* We've heard story after story about people who had previously been resigned to living life with their illnesses, conditions, or health concerns. These are people just like you who have had years of headaches, rashes, aches, and pains, and struggled with energy until they tried our soups. After they nourished their bodies with the highest-quality ingredients possible, the widest array of nutrients possible, and the freshest food possible, their symptoms disappeared, their dependence on medication waned, and their satisfaction with life skyrocketed. It stands to reason: Did you know that every medicine in science comes from some plant or something from nature?

Balance is the key. When one is in balance—eating well, sleeping well, hydrating, getting movement—the sky's the limit! We believe that many of us don't even know the potential our bodies are capable of. What if you fed your body the cleanest foods and had the ultimate rest and dealt with your stress in a healthy way? What could you accomplish? What could your body do? That's why our tag line is, "Body Pure, Mind Strong." Now that's sexy at any age!

OUR HEALTH COMMANDMENTS

To get you on the path to sexy, here are a few basic truths to know about your health—which also form the foundation of the Soupure philosophy and cleanse:

- **Health begins on the cellular level.** Healthy cells are made from healthy foods. Period.
- **The body knows how to heal itself.** Not only does the body know how to detoxify itself—which we'll talk about in just a bit—but it knows how to heal itself. All we need to do is give it the right tools to do it, stop giving it junk that hinders its function, and, well, get out of the way.
- **Take it back to our roots.** Today's processed and convenience foods wouldn't be recognizable to our grandparents or their grandparents. Foods that are rich in things like phytonutrients,

healthy fats, proteins, complex carbohydrates, minerals, and nutrients—whether in plant or animal form—are what the body was designed to live and thrive off of.

- **Go the extra mile.** Many diets encourage you to look back to what your ancestors ate in order to create healthier eating habits. We believe that's only partially helpful. The world is a very different place than it was a hundred, even fifty years ago. There are pesticides on our food, lead in our water, radiation in our air, and even toxins leaching into our food from plastic containers. We not only need to get back to traditional diet-based healing methods, we need to provide *extra* nourishment and support to protect our bodies from everything that's happening in our environments.

- **Food is information.** As Marlyn, our nutritionist, likes to say, "Every bite of food you eat is either adding to your health or depleting it. It can create a positive, healing environment, or it can trigger reactions that create damaging change in the body. We want to turn on the good stuff and turn off the bad."

- **The body is wise.** Your body knows what it's talking about. It can give you valuable feedback, if you're listening.

I have rosacea, and it's aggravated by certain foods. I've done three Soupure cleanses and each time my skin was noticeably better by the third day. That's just from doing the cleanse—eating soups all day. That's a really big deal.

—Debra M.

BALANCE REIGNS SUPREME

The body is always seeking balance—not too cold, not too hot, not too acidic, not too alkaline—so we should too. Right now the health dialogue is very black-or-white: Kale is good and carbs are bad! Fat is good and sugar is bad! Fat is bad and sugar is good! Raw is good and cooked is bad! We may never know what most of these debates will amount to, but we do know this: Too much of anything is not a good thing. Even too much water can kill you! So let's focus less on absolutes and more on getting healing food in and not-so-healing food out.

We also can't tell you how many times we hear, "Well, I've already blown my diet, so today is a wash. I'll be good tomorrow." We don't know how it happened, but people think that healthy eating needs to start first thing in the morning and continue all day or it doesn't count. Let tomorrow be right now! Any harm that you may have done with indulging in those pancakes or that slice of pizza isn't as big a deal if you're balancing it with healthier choices for the rest of the day.

The last thing we want you to think is that these cleanses or this "soup cleanse" way of life is all-or-nothing. That couldn't be further from the truth! Yes, making more healthy choices will ultimately add up to better health. But that doesn't mean you get kicked out of the club for making less-healthy choices every now and then. We all know what happens when you're told something's the forbidden fruit—you want it even more! Just eat right and in moderation. Your body will do the rest.

Consider these soups the ultimate get-healthy resource. You'll have amazing results if you follow the program in this book, but you don't have to be doing an official cleanse to reap their benefits. Adding a soup or two a day or maybe even a few soups a week will enhance your nutrition and make you feel and look better even if you keep the rest of your diet the same. Your body will feel and reap the rewards of those added nutrients and will thank you.

WE ARE HEREBY GRANTING YOU PERMISSION TO BE IMPERFECT

Perfection is paralysis. Don't get caught up in blowing off your cleanse because you "cheated" and had a bag of chips. Pick up right where you left off! Your body would much rather you kept on giving it those nourishing soups than a day's worth of junk. Your body doesn't care whether you do it "perfectly." It just cares that you do it. We encourage you to take this process day by day, or even better, meal by meal. What Soupure is all about, after all, is a *lifestyle*—one with loving boundaries.

We completely understand that anything new can feel foreign, overwhelming, and big. But moving out of your comfort zone is where the magic happens. And over time, it becomes part of the norm. That's why we've kept our program simple, so you can take baby steps to get to wherever it is you want to go. Eventually, all those little steps will add up! Be gentle with yourself, give it time, and be compassionate if you fall down or step off the path. Move on, heat up a soup, and give yourself some love.

Health is not about being perfect or just looking good for a reunion or wedding or the next big event. It's about the big picture and the lifestyle choices you make to get there and how you look and feel every day. It's less about skinny jeans than it is about having the stamina to play with your kids or grandkids. It's about having the energy to support your body, a positive mental outlook, and relationships that nourish you. Through this book, we'll show you how to get there.

3

The Soup Solution

So why soup? Well, soup is renowned as a common healing food across most, if not all, societies—whether it's congee (long-cooked rice porridge made with herbs) used by the Chinese, English beef tea sipped by the Victorians, or your grandmother's chicken noodle. In essence, soup is a predigested meal that aids in the absorption of nutrients, allowing the body not only to rest but also to allocate all its energy toward healing, regenerating, and restoring. It's why liquid diets and soups are the diet of choice in hospitals and recovery centers throughout the world (though we'd argue that ours are probably more delicious!). People don't realize that it is really hard to get the nutrients from whole foods because it takes so much work to extract them through chewing. Many of us are mindlessly eating—because we're multitasking, in a rush, or eating for emotional reasons—and we don't chew our food enough. (More about chewing in a bit.) What is so great about our soups is that the extraction of the nutrients is already done for you and all you have to do is enjoy them to reap the benefits.

When made with whole, well-sourced ingredients without any

additives, GMOs (see "What About GMOs?" on page 49), pesticides, herbicides, artificial colors or flavorings, or fillers, soups carry all the essentials for health: fiber, healthy fats, vitamins, antioxidants, and phytonutrients. These building blocks support your entire body, from your blood and organs to your digestive and immune systems and even your neurological function. Soup can make you smarter and boost your mood! (Seriously.)

Here are all the reasons why we believe soup to be a superior means of nourishing the body:

- **It's an easy way to get a ton of vegetables.** Chances are, you're currently not eating enough veggies. Most people aren't. And no, a pumpkin spice latte doesn't count. Also, it's easy to get stuck in a veggie rut, eating the same two or three go-to vegetables over and over. (We're looking at you, kale addicts.) You need more nutrients than from just those three foods. Soup is a great way not only to get many vegetables into your diet, but also to get many different types of vegetables, plus healing herbs and spices and potent superfoods. There are sixty different nutrients in a single day of our soup cleanse—yes, sixty!
- **It's doing the chewing for you.** Chewing is an essential part of the digestion process because by breaking down larger bits of food into smaller ones, you're helping your stomach metabolize what you eat. Not chewing enough means not getting all the nutritional components out of your food while also requiring your body to use more energy to break it down.

  Because blended soups contain foods that are broken down already, you can access all that nourishment without expending as much digestive energy. Blending breaks open the cells of our foods and releases all the nutrients in a way that our bodies can assimilate. Then, with the energy we saved, our bodies can focus on more important tasks like undertaking long-overdue repairs. So you can see why many of our soups are blended.

- **It's loading you up with way more nutrients than you would normally take in.** If you took all the ingredients in one of our soups and put them on your plate in whole food form, there's no way you'd finish them without getting full, especially if you were chewing like a champ (meaning at least thirty seconds per mouthful). Chances are you'd barely put a dent in your meal. While that's a testament to just how amazing chewing is for boosting your satiety, it's not doing anything for your nutritional bottom line. Soup offers a way to pack in all the nutrition your body needs in a much more efficient way.

- **It's a surefire fiber fix.** Your body loves fiber. It feeds the good bacteria in your gut, helps balance your blood sugar, keeps cholesterol in check, aids good digestion, and moves all the junk out of the trunk, naturally pulling out toxins with it as it goes. Plus, it helps you get fuller faster and aids with weight loss. But the average American consumes below the daily recommended minimum of 20 grams of fiber. That's creating the risk of developing conditions like heart disease, diabetes, diverticulitis, obesity, constipation, and certain cancers like colon cancer. That's where eating soup comes in. By blending foods in their whole form, you're getting a megadose of fiber with every serving of soup you eat. Our one-day cleanse has approximately 30 grams of fiber per day!

- **It's alkalizing.** As we talked about in the previous chapter, your body is always seeking an alkaline state. It's healthier for your joints, tissues, organs, and blood, and it's the key to fending off disease. Thanks to our soups' foundation of veggies, fruits, nuts, seeds, and legumes, drinking them is like giving your body a soothing alkaline antidote.

- **It's an enzyme boost.** Enzymes are proteins that ignite reactions in the body like a match. They're particularly crucial for digestion, helping your body break down what you've eaten into smaller, more manageable bits to absorb and use as nourishment. Enzymes also help regenerate your organs and chip in with general body-wide maintenance.[1] But in a normal diet, we don't get enough enzymes, so we're stretching our enzymes too thin. The ones that were maybe busy with repairing your liver or kidneys might be called into action after you ate that 24-ounce T-bone. When that happens, you're using your body's resources to digest food and taking away from its resources to rebuild. With our soups, though, you're providing your body with a much larger workforce of enzymes, and you aren't straining your digestive system with hard-to-digest foods.

■ **It's giving you *real* vitamins.** Walk down the aisle of any grocery store and you can see all the promises that manufacturers make: "Now with more vitamin C!" "Fortified with iron!" "Vitamin D added!" It sounds pretty good, especially because most people are deficient in these things. But what you're seeing are synthetic vitamins that are created in a lab, not derived in their purest state from plants themselves. Not only are these vitamin impostors far inferior to the real things, but they're often made from substances like tar and petroleum—so they're not just not good for you, they're *bad* for you. Of course, food manufacturers wouldn't have to add these things in if their products naturally contained them in the first place, making yet another strong case against eating processed foods. Vitamin supplements are also a lesser form of nutrients than their plant-derived counterparts. There's mounting evidence that getting the goods in pill form just isn't going to cut it, and it's definitely *not* giving you the benefits it's promising. In 2013, three studies were simultaneously published in *Annals of Internal Medicine*, each debunking commonly held beliefs about over-the-counter supplements (that they can prevent early death, stave off cognitive decline associated with aging, or help those who have had heart attacks prevent another one). An editorial accompanying these studies read, "Enough is enough.

Stop wasting money on vitamin and mineral supplements."[2] Bottom line: Your body thrives when you consume your nutrients from food.

Homemade soups have the real deal when it comes to vitamins. And because they contain a wide array of vitamins, you're getting everything the body needs from your food.

- ■ **It's easy.** The convenience is what first attracted us to soups— you can batch cook a few, freeze whatever's extra, and have meals that are quick to prepare and carry with you, whether it's for school lunches, running errands, or bringing to work.
- ■ **It's beauty food.** It bears repeating that soup can be very sexy. Since our versions are loaded with such a wide array of vitamins, minerals, and antioxidants, they can help you age more slowly and look more beautiful. A diet rich in essential nutrients can give you glowing skin, lustrous hair, and stronger nails.

While undergoing chemotherapy and radiation, my brother had no appetite and distaste for food at a time when nutrition was all-important. He found Soupure's chilled soups especially palatable. I was comforted by the knowledge that he was enjoying such nutritionally dense foods and maximizing his health as he fought cancer.

—Lillian K., MD

BONE BROTHS: NATURE'S MAGIC ELIXIR

Bone broths have been gaining in popularity lately, and for good reason. They have been used in traditional Chinese medicine for centuries to nourish the kidneys, fortify the blood, and support our vital essence (or chi). There's no fancy wizardry involved in making them, though: Bone broths are simply stocks made from animal bones. They evolved from a time when none of the animal went to waste, and traditional cultures understood that there were many healing benefits—in addition to delicious ones—from sipping this broth. Unfortunately, as the corner butcher store has been replaced with the corner fast-food restaurant, bone broths have started to become a thing of the past.

Cooking bones for hours and hours breaks down both the bones and the connective tissues, giving us proteins, minerals, and fat—all elements that heal in various ways. According to the Chinese medical theory that like supports like, bone tissue relates to the kidneys, which also govern the bones as well as the adrenals—which relate directly to immune health. Collagen, which is crucial for your bones, ligaments, cartilage, and brain, can even be effective in treating arthritis and other degenerative joint diseases. It's also a powerful antiaging remedy for your skin. Gelatin, a form of collagen, can help digestion. Bone marrow strengthens your immune system by carrying oxygen to cells in the body. Minerals such as calcium and phosphorus help maintain healthy bones and create energy in the body. There's emerging evidence that bone broth can also heal gut-related issues that many people suffer from, whether it's acid reflux,

As I am a doctor of traditional Chinese medicine, Soupure is definitely in line with my approach to healing. I often suggest warm, nutrient-dense foods to my patients to strengthen their digestion and nourish their bodies. I especially love Soupure's bone broth, which in Chinese medicine is used to boost the immune system and fortify the internal organs. I highly recommend these soups as a delicious and convenient way to supercharge your diet with vegetables, fruit, fiber, protein, and good fats!

—Cathy T., L.Ac., FABORM

ulcers, lactose or gluten intolerance (including celiac), diverticulitis, constipation, irritable bowel syndrome, or leaky gut. And now
experts suggest that healing the gut also means strengthening both
the immune and the neurological systems, making bone broth a
potent remedy for the entire body.[3] It's why we recommend starting
your day with a warm mug of healing broth, especially one you made
with love from the best ingredients possible.

SOUP VERSUS JUICE: WE'RE UNIM"PRESSED"

With a juice shop on every corner, you might think that cold-pressed
juice had all the answers. We get it! It's tempting to think we can
cure all of our ailments and complaints with what's in those attrac-
tive bottles. Plus, who doesn't love a refreshing glass of juice?

We're certainly not opposed to the occasional green juice. But let's
face it, cold juice that is void of fiber and protein is not a meal, so how
do you have a whole day of it and feel satisfied? Or nourished? Our
soups, on the other hand, are full of all the nutrition and sustenance
you need to not feel depleted or deprived. It's why we say, "Souping
is the new juicing." We don't think juice is necessarily bad if enjoyed
in moderation or as a supplement to your regular diet, but we do
believe—and doctors, nutritionists, and fitness experts agree (www
.soupure.com/testimonials/)—that our soups are a better way to
support the body. Here's why:

- **Foods like to be whole.** Plants, especially fruits and vegetables,
  hold a tremendous amount of nutrients in *all* of their bits and
  bobs—the peel, pulp, rind, seeds, and flesh. That's why we
  believe that all of it should go into our nourishing soups. But
  most important, using whole fruits and vegetables means getting every bit of their fiber.

- **Fiber is king.** As we mentioned above, fiber is essential to total health. So why throw it away?! Think about the little tray under your juicer after you've juiced some carrots, Swiss chard, or beets. That mound of stringy confetti? That's fiber! Not including it in the mix reduces most fruits and vegetables to simple sugars, which spike your blood sugar levels, leave your liver overworked, and imbalance your kidneys. Plus, when you dismantle a whole food, you're not getting all of its macronutrients, like protein and good fats. Without them, your body has a harder time absorbing other good stuff, rendering many vitamins and minerals unusable. Last, all that fiber is what's going to bind to the toxins in your system and pull them out of your intestinal tract and colon.
- **Some vegetables need cooking.** The body requires food in a variety of forms—raw and not raw—in order to feel optimally good. While eating raw food is necessary for good health, it's important for your absorption of plant protein and your nutrient diversity to include gently cooked food too. Read more about raw versus cooked food on page 35.
- **Don't get left in the cold.** According to ancient wisdom shared by traditional Chinese medicine and Ayurveda (Hindu medicine), warming foods are more healing, nourishing, and soothing to the body. They are the first real "comfort food" known to mankind. They also help stoke the digestive fire, which is at the center of your body's ability to break down and assimilate foods and all their nutrients. Having a lot of cold foods can put out that fire and dampen your digestion as well as your energy level. Just think about it: Would you rather have a day of cold liquid, or hearty, warm comfort food?

Above all, our favorite feature of souping is that it's not something you do *before* you start your diet. It *is* the diet! It's not something you have to get through in order to get to the next phase. It *is* the phase. It's a lifestyle that you can maintain forever and ever, because you're not starving and you're eating in a way that continuously supports the body. And it's easy enough to follow this program that souping won't disrupt all the other things you have going on in your busy life.

The Case for Cooked

Raw-food enthusiasts like to tout that by not heating their ingredients above 118°F, they're preserving even more of their nutritional benefits. However, we've learned that conservative cooking—like making a soup—actually makes most nutrients *more* absorbable. In fact, some nutrients can actually be *lost* if certain foods are eaten raw. According to an article by Joel Fuhrman, MD, gentle cooking can increase the plant proteins in your diet (extra-important if you're limiting animal foods), boost a plant's assimilation by destroying harmful antinutrients that can bind to certain minerals, reduce the amount of your own enzymes needed to break down food (saving your body precious energy), increase absorption of antioxidants, and allow your body to access more of the anticancer compounds found in plants.[4] Also, let's face it—sometimes nothing beats a warm bowl of chicken noodle soup.

Soupure soups are a godsend! They are the perfect antidote to recharge your nutritional intake and jump-start a healthier lifestyle. I am not a fan of cleanses usually, but I was intrigued by the Soupure concept. I did the three-day mini-cleanse and it was amazing. I was satisfied, didn't feel hungry, and I lost five pounds. Plus the soups are not only nutritious, they are delicious too. I find myself craving them! My coworker and I have decided to do a one-day cleanse each Monday as a way to kick our workweek into high gear. Thank you, Soupure!

—Leslie M.

Part II

READY, SET, GO!

4

Your New Pantry
Prescription

As you gear up for cleansing—and living your new and improved life afterward—it's important to understand just how powerful food is. Hippocrates wasn't kidding around when he said, "Let food be thy medicine and medicine be thy food."

Our soups are a way to help your body purify itself by flooding it with active, living macronutrients, micronutrients, live nutraceuticals, and enzymes. In a nutshell, these soups are like giving your body every miracle drug that nature invented. Unlike processed foods containing chemical additives and preservatives, which are suspected to cause fatigue, weight gain, gastrointestinal distress, and other ill effects that impact your longevity, our soups call for 100 percent fresh, unmanufactured, pesticide-free, non-GMO (see "What About GMOs?" on page 49), and fiber-rich ingredients not only to fight the adverse effects of an increasingly toxic world, but also to protect you from health insults down the road.

So no matter if you want to lose weight, heal from an injury or surgery, boost your libido, find a new sense of calm, or just beat the common cold—there's a soup for you! That's not because we're some kind of soup wizards; it's because that's simply how food works. Soups, though, are only as good as the foods you put in them—and that's where we come in. We've figured out how to harness the natural goodness of a whole host of foods—and lots of *super*foods—and combine them in the most delicious, satisfying way possible. We worked hard to determine what nutrients and vitamins most people are missing in their diets and made sure to include them on our soup roster.

Think of this book as a prescription for health, your pantry and fridge as your new medicine cabinets, and the food you put into your body as your new medication. Every single whole, healthy food you eat is giving you all the tools you need for immune health, digestive wellness, mental strength and clarity, hormonal balance, libido heightening, and emotional enhancement. And while we know that beauty isn't just skin deep, it doesn't hurt that these foods also contribute to looking slim and sexy, and all-around radiating with health.

To give you an idea of just how essential getting a wide array of vegetables, fruits, seeds, nuts, legumes, spices, and herbs is, we included a small glossary below of the almost-too-good-to-be-true benefits of just some of our ingredients. And the best news? Every single one of these can be found in our recipes in chapter 11. Check out that section for even more information about the superpowers of food.

Almonds

- Help in brain development
- Regulate cholesterol levels
- Fortify the heart
- Improve complexion

Bananas

- Reduce menstrual pains
- Settle an upset digestive system
- Lower the risk of kidney cancer

Beets

- Help maintain strong bones
- Lower blood pressure
- Boost sex hormones
- Reduce cancer risk

Brazil nuts

- Prevent heart disease
- Reduce cancer risk
- Boost liver health

Carrots

- Improve vision
- Help clear acne
- Reduce risk of stroke and cancer

Coconut

- Contains antibacterial properties
- Is naturally hydrating
- Boosts energy and metabolism

Dates

- Help cure intestinal disorders
- Increase stamina
- Fortify the heart

Flaxseeds

- Balance hormones
- Stabilize blood sugar levels
- Regulate cholesterol levels
- Promote fertility

Garbanzo beans (chickpeas)

- Increase satiety
- Regulate blood sugar
- Provide digestive support

Garlic

- Improves iron absorption
- Promotes heart health
- Has anti-inflammatory properties

Ginger

- Aids digestion
- Alleviates allergies
- Prevents and treats colds and flus
- Lowers cholesterol

Lemons

- Have antibacterial properties
- Fight wrinkles and blackheads
- Reduce mental stress and depression

Lentils

- Boost heart health
- Improve circulation
- Aid in energy production and metabolism

Mint

- Relieves respiratory disorders
- Improves skin conditions
- Reduces cancer risk
- Has antibacterial properties

Onion

- Promotes heart health
- Has anti-inflammatory properties
- Supports bone and connective tissue health

Pineapple

- Helps maintain strong bones
- Aids in digestion
- Prevents and treats the common cold

Spinach

- Helps bone maintenance
- Lowers blood pressure
- Protects against eye disease
- Reduces cancer risk

Strawberries

- Fight inflammation
- Reduce cancer risk
- Lower blood pressure

Sunflower seeds

- Strengthen bones
- Boost heart health

Turmeric

- Reduces cancer risk
- Stabilizes blood sugar levels
- Aids in liver detoxification
- Acts as a natural pain reliever

Vanilla bean

- Contains disease-fighting antioxidants
- Acts as a potent aphrodisiac
- Reduces cancer risk
- Has soothing and soporific properties

From the Nutritionist: Marlyn Diaz, CN

I've been involved in the nutrition, health, and food industry for over twenty-five years. Before I knew I wanted to help people take control of their wellness through diet—before I even had a job—I innately knew there was a connection between food and health. I wrote my first term paper in the tenth grade, back in the 1970s, on food additives and the correlation between the MSG in Chinese takeout I'd eat and the headaches I'd get. This sense that what I put in my body affected how it was able to function has since informed my approach to health. When I dealt with my own health challenges in my twenties—chronic fatigue syndrome, digestive challenges, hormonal imbalance—I looked beyond conventional medicine and found doctors who understood that wellness starts on a cellular level and that food is information for the body.

Ever since, I've been studying how some foods damage the body, while others heal it. What I've come to understand is this: *The blood of a plant nourishes the blood of a human.* Sure, plants don't have blood the way we think of it, but they do have a life source: chlorophyll. And just as plants get their health and energy from the sun, we get our health and energy from plants. When we chew a stalk of asparagus or munch some Brussels sprouts, we crack open those plants' cells and flood our body with all the nutrients that they have to offer. And by extension, we alkalize our systems, reduce inflammation, bring balance, and promote healing. These foods were designed by nature to nourish the body.

When it comes to *how* to eat plants, I tell my clients to "eat the rainbow." By eating all the colors that exist in the plant world, you can guarantee that you're getting tons of minerals, vitamins, nutrients, and other powerful compounds that are cancer-fighting and detoxifying. Think about the red of a tomato, the orange of a bell pepper, the yellow of a summer squash, the green of broccoli, the blue of blueberries, and the purple of an eggplant—each distinct color is advertising that plant's unique phytochemical powers. One of the reasons why I love these soups so much is because they're a no-brainer way of getting in so much nutrition.

WILL I GET ENOUGH PROTEIN WITH PLANTS?

While we're not strict vegetarians, we both believe in the power of plants and their protein. Let's dive in a bit deeper here. Animal proteins (like chicken, steak, and fish) are known to be complete proteins, while plant proteins (such as those in broccoli, spinach, and kale) are incomplete. The term "complete protein" refers to the amino acids that make up the protein, the building blocks of the human body. There are nine essential amino acids that the body can't produce on its own, which is where complete-protein foods come into play.[1]

While plants don't have every single one of these amino acids, advocates of veganism and vegetarianism claim that humans don't need every essential amino acid in every meal and that plant-based diets contain enough variety to give us a sufficient amount of amino acids every day.[2] We believe that with a balanced, well-rounded diet composed primarily of plants, you're going to get the protein you need. For those of you who eat meat—and we think that animal foods are a beneficial addition to the diet in moderation—then you're absolutely covering your bases. These foods are complete proteins and also provide nutrients like B_{12} and carnitine, essential fatty acids, and certain fat-soluble vitamins, which are harder to get from a plant-based diet.

THE END OF COUNTING CALORIES

For years, counting calories was considered the key to maintaining a healthy weight. We remember torturing ourselves over every single little one, not even really understanding what exactly a calorie is and whether it truly holds the secrets to a trimmer waistline or improved wellness. In scientific terms, a calorie is a unit of energy. So when you hear something described as having 100 calories, that's how much energy your body gains from that food. While calories aren't intrinsically bad for you—your body needs them for energy—not all calories are created equal. That's why we believe that you should, once and for all, *stop counting calories.*

The biggest reason for ditching the calorie tally is that not all calories make you fat. "Empty calories," or calories derived from processed carbohydrates and alcohols, not only lead to weight gain but are completely devoid of nutrients such as vitamins, minerals, antioxidants, amino acids, or dietary fiber. Think cake, cookies, sweets, soft drinks, beer, wine, and other spirits, as well as many savory processed foods like salad dressings, breads, tomato sauces, and crackers that sneak added sugars into your diet. On the other hand, calories that come from whole, nourishing foods give your body the energy it needs while being utilized in a totally different way. Calories from plants—such as fruits, vegetables, grains, nuts, and legumes—get put to good and efficient use in the body, compared to empty calories, which get stored as fat. So instead of looking at the number of calories on, say, a Kit Kat bar and one of our soups, think about comparing what those calories are doing for you and how each makes you look and feel. We encourage you to ditch the calorie dogma and simply listen to how your body feels when it's eating real food.

DOES ORGANIC MATTER?

Some people think that the organic label is just a marketing scam, while others live and die by it. Who is right? At Soupure, we tell people that our soups are made with over 90 percent organic ingredients. Does that mean that we ran out of steam after finding the best ingredients and threw in 10 percent of junk? Not even close. We strive to use only organic ingredients whenever possible. But, truth be told, sometimes—like the average health-conscious consumer— we cannot find, for example, that organic cinnamon to complete our soup. If it's an ingredient we're using in a small amount, we might go non-organic, or we'll get our produce locally sourced if it means better quality even if it's missing the organic label. It turns out that official organic certification is expensive, and some farmers, no matter how much loving care they put into their soil, can't afford it. So they can't technically say that their wares are organic, even though they're probably ten times healthier than what you'd find anywhere else.

What this taught us is that we need to look a little deeper than labels, which we'll admit can get a little confusing. We also don't love the idea of absolutes. We are, after all, about balance. That includes grocery shopping. So here's a little primer on how to get the best food in a way that's most convenient for you:

- **Organic is better than conventional.** When you buy "Certified Organic," it means that you are buying something grown in healthy soil nourished with nothing but organic matter—no pesticides, herbicides, or other nasty chemicals. It's not only better for the planet but also better for you since plants grown in organic soil have been shown to develop more antioxidants than conventional plants. The same rule of thumb applies to animal products (i.e., meat and bones): "Certified Organic" denotes animals that are raised in a responsible way with a biologically correct (non-GMO—see "What About GMOs?" on page 49 for more information) diet, no hormones, and no antibiotics. This means a healthier animal, and ultimately a healthier you.

- **When in doubt, buy local.** Since food grown in your area doesn't have to be shipped halfway around the world, it tends to be less expensive than organic foods brought in from another continent. Even though some smaller farming operations can't afford an official organic certification, they are less likely to spray their crops with heavy-duty industrial chemicals. If you shop at a farmers' market, all you have to do is ask. The best way to learn about your farmers' practices is to meet them face-to-face. We love our farmers' markets!

- **In a pinch, learn the list.** If you can't afford to buy all organic or don't have access to a variety of organic produce, at least you can avoid what the Environmental Working Group has dubbed the "Dirty Dozen Plus"—those conventionally grown foods that consistently test high for pesticide residue, including:

Apples	Nectarines
Celery	Peaches
Cherry tomatoes	Potatoes
Cucumbers	Snap peas (imported)
Grapes	Spinach
Hot peppers	Strawberries
Kale/collard greens	Sweet bell peppers

Conversely, you could buy the "Clean Fifteen," the conventionally raised fruits and vegetables that test lowest for pesticide residue so you don't need to worry about whether or not they are organic:

Asparagus	Cabbage
Avocados	Cantaloupe

Cauliflower

Eggplant

Grapefruit

Kiwi

Mangoes

Onions

Papaya

Pineapples

Sweet corn

Sweet peas (frozen)

Sweet potatoes

Unfortunately, the deceivingly simple "thick-skinned theory" doesn't hold up. We used to think that thick-skinned fruit such as pineapples, bananas, and citrus didn't need to be organic because it would eventually be peeled. But it turns out that some pesticides and herbicides can penetrate produce's skin, which is pretty scary because these chemicals have been associated with health problems such as non-Hodgkin's lymphoma and reproductive dysfunction.[3]

WHAT ABOUT GMOs?

GMOs, or genetically modified organisms, are foods whose genetic material has been artificially manipulated by a process called genetic engineering, or GE. This practice is mainly used so a crop can withstand even more herbicides and/or insecticides (meaning a GM food you bring home has been sprayed with that much more!). There's significant emerging research that connects GMOs with health problems, including digestive issues and reproductive disorders.[4]

Even though the United States has approved GMOs, we take our cue from the more than sixty countries around the world—including Australia, Japan, and the entire European Union—that do not consider GMOs to be safe and have either restricted or banned their sale.

The easiest way to avoid GMOs is to buy organic, as no food labeled "Certified Organic" can be GM. Otherwise, here's a list of the most common GM foods and substances in the United States:

- Aspartame
- Canola oil
- Corn
- Milk (in dairy cow feed)
- Papaya
- Soy
- Sugar
- Yellow squash
- Zucchini[5]

ORGANIC AND PACKAGED FOODS

You have to be vigilant when buying any food that has been processed, packaged, and decorated with a label. Food manufacturers love making all kinds of claims to seduce you into buying their product, whether it's promises like "Farm Fresh," "All Natural," or "Pure," or pictures of sunny fields or bucolic orchards. Here's the scoop: The only label that carries official oversight is "USDA Organic." There's no standardized meaning for those other terms, which means manufacturers can promise the world but still sneak in any number of additives. That said, organic processed foods aren't always as good as they seem, either. Organic nut milks, for example, frequently contain things like xanthan gum, soy lecithin, and carrageenan, which have been linked to a number of detrimental health effects.[6] Bottom line: Read labels and be wary of any ingredient you wouldn't keep in your pantry.

SUPER ADD-INS

While all plants are pretty super in our book, there are some foods that go above and beyond the call of duty. These potent soup add-ins are typically very concentrated and found in far-flung nooks of the globe, which can make them a tad more pricey than run-of-the-mill fruits and vegetables. But we promise that investing in these ingredients will pay back in spades—they're your new healing remedies!

Don't feel like you have to go out and buy them all at once, though. Try to build up a collection over time. Choose one or two from this list each time you go grocery shopping, or perhaps every other trip, to help spread out the cost. In just a few weeks or months you'll have a pantry stocked with some of the most powerful ingredients on the planet. And you will use them in no time—start with our soups and expand to your own recipes! If you don't have a great health food store or organic grocer near you, it's easy to find these items online.

- **Cordyceps.** This powder made from mushrooms is prized among athletes for stimulating athletic performance, overall stamina, and immune response.
- **Reishi powder.*** The powder of these gorgeous East Asian fungi is one of the oldest substances in Chinese medicine; it has been used for over two thousand years to treat the body with its divine powers. It contains the rare ganoderic acid that is shown to have antibacterial and antiviral properties, and may also inhibit tumor growth.
- **Maca root.*** Grown in the high plateaus of the Andes in Peru, this relative of the radish helps boost the libido, balance hormones, and enhance your palate with its hint of butterscotch taste.
- **Raw honey.** In addition to being nature's delicious sweetener, raw honey is a powerful antimicrobial, antiviral, and antifungal agent, as well as an antioxidant. The phytonutrients found in honey have also been shown to possess cancer-preventing and antitumor

---

* While these noted ingredients are amazingly beneficial, they can be contra-indicated for women who are pregnant or nursing. Consult with your health care practitioner before adding them to your diet.

properties. Not all honey is created equal, though. Be sure to buy one that is raw—processed honey has lost most of its nutritional value—and from a reputable (organic if possible) producer.

- **Maple syrup.** Maple is a mineral powerhouse, with substantially more manganese, riboflavin, and zinc, and less sugar per unit, than honey.
- **Dried apricots.** Rich in soluble fiber, dried apricots provide a plant gel specially designed to bind with excess fats during digestion and remove them from the body efficiently. Also a significant source of iron, they not only work to prevent clogging of the arteries, but also boost your red blood cells' ability to attract oxygen.
- **Chia seeds.** Dating back to ancient Mayan and Aztec societies, chia are an edible desert seed known to curb the appetite and provide an unusually high concentration of protein, fat, fiber, carbohydrates, minerals, and vitamins. They also contain age-defying antioxidants and help lower cholesterol and maintain strong bones.
- **Miso.** Miso, or fermented soybean paste, has been a staple in Chinese and Japanese diets for approximately twenty-five hundred years. Today, most of the Japanese population starts their day with a warm bowl of miso soup believed to stimulate digestion and energize the body. Miso also contains all the essential amino acids, making it a complete protein; stimulates the secretion of digestive fluids in the stomach; restores beneficial probiotics to the intestines; strengthens the quality of the blood and lymph fluid; reduces the risk for breast, prostate, lung, and colon cancers; protects against radiation; strengthens the immune system; lowers cholesterol; and is high in antioxidants that protect against free radicals. Phew!

Though soy can be difficult to digest, fermenting it changes the way the body can assimilate its nutrients. That makes for an enormous difference between live-enzyme miso and soy chips. Just make sure you buy a non-pasteurized version, which you can find in the refrigerated case at the grocery store.

- **Dandelion tea.** Used for many generations as an herbal medicinal, dandelion tea is known to decrease swelling. Often used as a gentle diuretic, it breaks down fat and toxins in the liver and assists the organs with their blood-cleansing duties.

THE MOST IMPORTANT INGREDIENT: WATER

Over half of your body is made up of water, which is a pretty good reason to keep hydrated. But water is also essential for helping the body detoxify. The cells have their own detoxification system, so they're always releasing toxins, chemicals, and the aftermath of cellular function into the bloodstream. Water helps flush that out. Also, since many of us are walking around in a more acidic state thanks to stress or diet or lifestyle, the body is constantly trying to do damage control, and a lot of that detoxification is also ending up in the blood. That's why we recommend drinking two cups of water first thing in the morning—imagine that the janitors came at night to sweep up, and now the trash needs to go out. Plus, your body is naturally more dehydrated in the morning. So wake up, drink some water, pee, poop, and drink some more water—get the junk out and put the good stuff in. Plus, you'll be well on your way toward proper hydration. (This goes double for you coffee drinkers—have water before and after your coffee.) Water is also important for brain health, so if you're not thinking clearly or feel foggy, drink some water. It's the elixir of life!

Luckily, eating a diet that's rich in plants is a great way to meet your water goal. But drinking plenty of water is necessary too. We recommend taking your body weight and dividing it in half to compute the number of ounces you should drink in a day. For example, if you weigh 120 pounds, then you should be drinking 60 ounces. Sometimes we hear that people don't love the taste of water. That's why we include three of our delicious, easy-to-make (not to mention beautiful to look at) infused alkaline water recipes in chapter 10. Herbal tea is a nice way to hydrate too; just try not to add processed sugar or artificial sweeteners.

Keep in mind that if you're actively dehydrating the body—exercising, drinking coffee or alcohol—then you need to drink even more water. The rule of thumb is definitely true: If you're feeling thirsty, then you're already dehydrated. And sometimes when you're feeling hungry, you're really just thirsty. Try to catch dehydration before it happens—which should no longer be a chore with yummy infused alkaline waters!

As for what kind of water, we'll keep it simple: the purest you can get. Ideally you can drink at least some alkaline water. You can buy an alkaline filter or buy an alkaline water pitcher at Costco or Office Depot, and retailers like Wal-Mart, Whole Foods, and Gelson's all carry alkaline water in bottles for sale. Drinking alkaline water boosts your energy and your metabolic rate, rebuilds your immune system, and helps your body absorb vitamins and nutrients more efficiently. In essence, your vital organs function their best in an alkaline environment, and drinking alkaline water supports that goal. It's an easy way to help keep your body clean and operating at peak performance. That's why we use it as the foundation for our infused waters, which we recommend sipping frequently throughout your day—especially during a cleanse.

WHAT'S ALL THE FUSS OVER "GOOD FATS" VERSUS "BAD FATS"?

You'll notice that a few of our recipes call for a decent amount of fat, whether it's from nuts and seeds or olive oil. But here's the thing:

Fat doesn't make you fat. As you read in chapter 2, eating processed foods, refined sugar, and an otherwise imbalanced diet made up of poor-quality foods is what makes you gain weight.

Without fat, your body can't use many of the critical vitamins and minerals you consume, like vitamins A, E, and D. Fat surrounds every cell membrane of your body so it can metabolize. Fat lines your nerves to send signals and reflexes faster between your brain and body. Fat regulates your hormones and your body temperature. Fat protects all of your most vital organs from injury. Fat is efficient brain food that allows signals to speed along. It also makes your skin and hair beautiful, touchable, and sexy. Say it with us: Fats are good for you.

So don't skip the fat to stay fit. Nature intended it to serve as the best mechanism to help us survive on this planet, perpetuate our families, and give us a sense of well-being. That's why we have incorporated the right ratio of good fats into our soup recipes from sources like hearty nuts, yummy seeds, energizing coconut, and rich extra-virgin olive oil.

Fats in a Nutshell

"Good" fats. High in omega-3s, these are also known as essential fatty acids. We need to get them from outside sources, as the body does not manufacture its own. Hence the word "essential." We can get them from vegetables, nuts, seeds, and fish.

"Bad" fats. These include trans fats and saturated fats, including fats from margarine, butter, fats used in deep frying, oils that have been used in processed foods, hydrogenated oils, fats that have high amounts of omega-6s like soybean oil, and most processed vegetable oils. They raise your bad cholesterol (the kind that clogs up your arteries) and lead to inflammation, which increases the risk for disease.

SHOULD I BE CONCERNED ABOUT SUGAR IN THE SOUPS?

Right now there's controversy over how much sugar you should have in a day and whether it's okay to eat sugar that comes from fruits and vegetables. Here's what we do know: Fruit and vegetable diets are *not* creating chronic disease. When you eat foods in their whole form, you're getting their sugar, but you're also getting their fiber, which binds to the sugars and makes for much gentler integration in the body. If we use any sweeteners in our soups, we opt for natural sugars in their whole state. These aren't just sweet and delicious, they're healing too. Moderate amounts of maple syrup, raw honey, dates, and dried apricots provide the taste you're looking for without overloading your system with sugar and setting you up for a crash.

PUTTING IT TOGETHER

Now that you have a clear idea of what's going to nourish your body and restore it to its optimal health, it's time to talk about *how* we're going to get there. How can you give your body the space it needs to repair, rebuild, and restore? How can you rev up your organs, tissues, and blood and keep them working at their optimal ability? In short: It's time for a cleanse.

5

Taking the Junk Out of the Trunk: Cleansing

Souping is the best way to balance and reset the body, while streamlining my lifestyle and waist. I love starting every day with an alkaline water to bring down the naturally occurring acidic levels of the body, and then a bone broth to clear and set up the gut/ digestive system for taking advantage of the healthy foods I'll be consuming throughout the rest of the day. Also, the soups just taste good. Since I started soup cleansing, I have experienced no more bloating or indigestion, less oily skin, cleaner pores, more radiant skin, and even shinier hair. Soupure has changed my everyday life for the better and encouraged a more conscientious way of living in my household, and it certainly can in yours.

—Michael F.

Our cleanse is a comprehensive way to help your body reset its natural rhythms. We aren't forcing your body to unnaturally flush itself through starvation. We are using food to assist your body in its natural cleansing process. Normally, your body needs to digest food, and digestion takes energy. So if your energy is going toward other events in life—whether it's negative like the stress of work or positive like doing activities you enjoy—your body might not have the bandwidth to properly break down that food. And when that happens, all that nutrition isn't being reaped or properly allocated to the parts of the body that need it most. That's why soups are such a beautiful thing.

By inundating your cells with every nutrient they need while simultaneously allowing your digestive system to rest and naturally expel its waste through its healthy organs, soups allow your body to focus its energy on healing itself and making bigger strides in building strength. Plus, giving your body a break from irritants and toxins means finally giving it the space to return to how it truly wants to be: balanced, calm, and resilient. It's a gentle enough process that, with the endorsement of physicians and oncologists, we've been able to offer our soups to patients undergoing chemotherapy who are on a liquid diet.

With our recipes, you'll be able to enjoy all the healthy benefits of whole fruits and vegetables, including their nutrition-packed skins, seeds, and rinds. Unlike liquid juice cleanses based on high-sugared fruits that can lead to spiked blood sugar and the inevitable energy crash, our cleanse offers the entire spectrum of flavor profiles from sweet to savory, and because we're using the whole plant, their nutrients are delivered to your body in a gentler way that your organs can handle. This is also great for cleansing because all that fiber is a key component of the detoxification process, naturally binding and whisking away all the bad stuff from your system. Fiber also aids effortless weight loss in the sound manner recommended by the medical community. And because we call for cooking certain foods—especially those that are more difficult for the body to break down and reap nourishment from—you'll be giving your body a rest while making the good stuff more digestible and absorbable.

The words "cleansing" and "detoxing" might make it sound like you'll be deprived, but unlike a juice cleanse, master cleanse, or any other "starvation cleanse," we're putting food and nourishment into the body. Simply put, liquid diets don't build your body. Our soups, however, nurture and support all your systems while still providing plenty of energy for you to get through your hectic day. There's no need to take time off from your normal life to do our program. You're eating *actual food* all day long! It's just being delivered in a way that gives your body space for rest and healing.

When is a good time to cleanse? Just about any time: if you want to boost your energy; when you want to lose weight; if you're about to have surgery and want to allow your body to be at its most efficient; when you're healing after surgery or an injury; to create a gateway to healthier eating; or if you have an event coming up that you want to look your absolute best for. Whatever the reasoning, we promise that by the end of the cleanse, you will feel better than you ever imagined. And because you have not starved yourself to get there, it should be

What Are Some of the Results I Might See After Cleansing?

You can look forward to looking and feeling better after finishing our cleanse! Here are some positive changes you may notice:

Better bowel function

Decreased gastrointestinal problems

Dissipation of chronic symptoms

Healthier skin and hair

Improved mood

Less inflammation

More energy and less fatigue

Organ support and regeneration

Weight loss and bloat reduction

easier for you to maintain the benefits you have achieved after your program is completed.

Just make sure, if appropriate, that you've checked with your doctor first if you plan on cleansing. The information provided here should not be used as a substitute for a physician's consultation, advice, or treatment. While our soups are powerful healers and should benefit all as real food, it's always advised that you work with your health care provider to ensure you're going to get everything you need in a way that's right for your own body.

You don't need a specific reason to start our cleanse—and you can have any number of motivations. But here are our personal favorite reasons for cleansing:

- **It gives your body a rest.** It takes a lot of energy to break down food. A soup cleanse gives the body a break from doing that while still nourishing every bit of you with nutrient-dense foods like vegetables, fruits, nuts, and seeds.
- **It gives you a clean slate.** Cleansing is the perfect way to reset your nutrition. Whether you're ready to make a lifestyle overhaul, have been indulging in one too many cheat days, or just aren't feeling top-notch, a few days of soups is what your body needs to scrub down, clean out, and prepare for better, brighter days ahead.
- **It's part of the natural order.** If you have pets, notice what they do when they're not feeling their greatest—they fast! Most animals, domesticated and in the wild, know to give their systems a break when their bodies need to heal. Cleansing is a potent double whammy—it allows you to rest your digestion while simultaneously flooding it with nutrients, which is giving your body all the tools it needs to restore itself.
- **It can help break a weight-loss plateau.** If you're trying to lose weight but keep hitting a wall, cleansing can give your body the nudge it needs. A cleanse tricks the body by not giving it the same old foods day after day, thus allowing it to recalibrate its systems.

For five years I have struggled with my weight and all sorts of diets. My doctor told me I was pre-diabetic and my cholesterol and glucose levels were in danger zones and wanted to put me on medication. I knew I had to lose weight and change my eating. Part of my problem is work. I leave early in the morning to work all day and eat unhealthy foods. It is so hard to find healthy fast food. I have tried more diets than I can remember. I would start to lose weight and only end up feeling miserable, and felt like I was starving myself. I was never satisfied and, even worse, after going off a diet I would gain back more weight than I had lost, in half the time.

I was so frustrated, but then I heard about Soupure. I love soup, so I was excited about the idea of a soup cleanse. When I looked into it and realized I could have eight products a day that were fast and easy to bring with me and eat, I decided to try the five-day cleanse. I lost four and a half pounds over the five days! I was so thrilled with the results, I consulted with my doctor about the nutritional value of Soupure, and we crafted a long-term souping plan for me.

I am not starving anymore! I eat multiple times a day and feel satisfied and full. I was always so busy with work that finding time to buy or prepare healthy food was not an option. With Soupure, I grab my bottles of soup, bring them to work or drink them in the car when I am driving. I can't believe that I don't feel hungry anymore. When I crave sweets, I have a cold soup and it takes care of those sugar cravings. I have lost 32 pounds and 5 inches from my waistline in a four-month period and I'm still going strong.

I feel so much better and my doctor cannot believe the improvements in my blood work and overall health. I am still going, and feeling so much better and healthier has given me the strength to finally quit smoking after at least seven previous attempts.

—Charlie W.

CLEANSE AT A GLANCE

Whether you choose a one-day, three-day, three-day mini, or five-day cleanse—which we'll talk more about in the next chapter—the rhythm of your day stays the same. You're going to be getting the same kind of nourishment in a sequence that works with your body's natural rhythms. This way you're not only getting all the nutrients you need, you're also getting them in a way that maximizes how your body can use them. While the soups will vary from day to day—because who wants to eat the same thing over and over again?—we have a variety of flavors and types that accomplish the same goals.

Here's what your routine will look like while soup cleansing—no starvation to be worried about here! If you're planning to be more active during your cleanse or are nervous about not having enough to eat (though you'd be surprised!), read on to the next chapter, where we address how to tailor this sequence to your needs.

- **Morning starter.** Start the day with 16 ounces of room-temperature water, either plain with a squeeze of fresh lemon juice or a flavored alkaline water (pages 112–115). The idea is you're doing a micro-cleanse to flush out what's been built up in the digestive tract overnight, mucus accumulation, and anything else the body has been repairing and detoxing overnight. Citrus fruits actually have the ability to penetrate your cells and push out toxins without using any of the body's energy, and once ingested they're also incredibly alkalizing and hydrating. Make sure you're drinking your water at room temperature, because cold water can be hard on the spleen and digestive system.
- **Hot morning chaser.** Broths (pages 140–146) are healing for the gut, especially when eaten on an empty stomach. That way you're receiving all the nutrients, instead of using them to

digest other food. Some of our broths include a dose of miso, which is a probiotic, full of enzymes, and a complete protein. It also has the ability to detox heavy metals and radiation. Our broths also call for kombu, a sea vegetable, which is rich in iodine—a necessary and balancing element for the body—and is also helpful in detoxing heavy metals. But ultimately it's a kind way to warm up the body in the morning and get it ready for the day to come.

- **Chilled breakfast or post-workout.** Called our Superhero (page 151), this chilled blend of seeds, nuts, and superfoods provides the omega fats, both 3 and 6, that you need for the day, and tastes like a delicious smoothie. It gives you the perfect essential fatty acid ratio balance, which is good for heart health, brain health, cholesterol, inflammation, and providing energy. You get a hit of zinc, which is an antioxidant that helps with healing related to stress on the body, as well as selenium, which is key for brain chemistry. Change it up with any of our other nut milks (pages 147–152). We recommend drinking these "soups" in the morning because they rev up your metabolism. Your body always has a choice about whether to get its energy from fat or from carbohydrates, and because you haven't had any carbohydrates yet, it's going to start dipping into your fat stores—and that's a good thing! If you are allergic to nuts, you should substitute our Superhero or other nut milks with a Cucumber-Grape-Honeydew Chilled Soup (our Refresh) (page 116); or Pineapple, Papaya, and Fennel Cold Soup (our Breathe) (page 117).

- **Hot lunch.** Lunch will often be a hot, veggie-based soup that incorporates olive oil (pages 120–140). That's so you can access all those fat-soluble vitamins in the soup like A, E, and D. As we mentioned earlier, you need that fat to really absorb these vitamins. You're also getting all the fiber from the veggies, which will be doing a clean sweep of your colon and will help you feel nice and full. As your body breaks down the vegetables, you'll not only get all their vitamins, but you'll also be feeding the microflora in your gut. Plus, having a hot soup is soothing and comforting—this is a part of the day you'll really enjoy.

- **Chilled afternoon snack.** A cold, fruit-based "soup" (pages 115–120) offers a quick hit of glucose and fructose to give you some energy and keep you from sneaking off to the vending machine for that pack of Twizzlers.
- **Hot dinner.** Just like lunch, dinner is a hot, vegetable-based soup with just enough healthy fat to absorb all the nutrients (pages 120–140). The soups we recommend for dinner often include a legume like lentils or a starchy vegetable like sweet potato, so you'll feel sated, content, and ready to get a good night's sleep.
- **Nightcap.** Some of our cleansers choose to add a veggie broth to the end of their day as a soothing treat to calm the body. Or if you're in the mood for something sweet, make a mug of one of our lattes or teas, such as Sweet Dreams (page 153).

In addition to your daily soup menu, we also highly recommend sipping herbal, decaffeinated teas and infused alkaline waters throughout the day to keep you balanced and hydrated. There's also the option to add small snacks in a pinch, which we'll talk more about in chapter 7.

DIGGING IN

Excited to start your cleanse? We know we are! We can't wait for you to experience this incredible transformation, free from deprivation or hunger. You'll wish someone had told you sooner about just how delicious and satisfying cleansing could be!

6

Choosing and Preparing for Your Cleanse

Whether you're an expert detoxer or a nervous first-timer, there's absolutely a cleanse for you. Here's how to choose which cleanse is right for you:

One-Day Cleanse

For you if:

- The only veggies you eat are what comes on your burger.
- The word "detox" still gives you the willies.
- You're a pro at detoxing and just want weekly maintenance after finishing a five-day. (We highly recommend the one-day maintenance cleanse. And there's nothing like a once-a-week mini-cleanse to keep everything running smoothly.)

Three-Day Cleanse

For you if:

- You've flirted with "health food" but aren't in a committed relationship.
- You're an adventuresome detox newbie.
- You have a reunion/wedding/gala/special event this weekend and want to look amazing.
- You're trying to kick a bug. You know the saying "feed a cold"? Well, there is nothing better than a day of our nourishing soups to help heal your cold, cough, or minor illness.

Three-Day Mini-Cleanse

This program differs from our full three-day cleanse in that you supplement a solid-food meal for either lunch or dinner, your choice. We've provided recipe suggestions for potential meal supplements in chapter 11.

For you if:

- You've conquered the one-day but aren't ready for the three-day plunge.
- You're new to cleansing but are ready for a challenge.
- Your schedule makes it hard to have soups for every meal.
- You want to incorporate soups into your everyday diet but want to get in some good old-fashioned chewing too.

Five-Day Cleanse

For you if:

- You're new to cleansing but have no fear—let the healing begin!
- You're experiencing uncomfortable symptoms and want to give your body room to take care of business.

- You've kicked all kinds of detox butt and are looking to take it to a new level.
- You have a long road of weight loss and improved eating habits ahead and want a big jump-start.

For Extra Credit

To really ensure that you're firing on all cylinders, we recommend this long-term cleansing program:

- A one-day cleanse once a week to regularly reset your systems.
- A three-day cleanse once a month.
- A five-day cleanse whenever you're feeling heavy or sluggish or in need of a reboot.

Doing a Soupure cleanse is like being at a funky restaurant that only serves the most unbelievable soups and smoothies. Each one is better than the next. I managed to feel totally satisfied—even while facilitating a field trip for second-graders and watching them eat In-N-Out Burger.

—Tabitha S.

HOW WILL I FEEL DURING A CLEANSE?

Detoxing (or in our case, "eating clean") isn't always easy. It's a change. It can be simple and smooth for some, while for others there might be a withdrawal effect of coming off foods like sugar, alcohol, and caffeine. If you're already eating clean, then this will most likely be a very easy transition. From our experience, most people feel a sense of "lightness" in their body and mind and a boost of energy—especially because they're not starving themselves!

If you are someone who is used to a diet that includes a lot of heavy meats, processed foods, sugar, caffeine, and alcohol, you want to wean off of these foods several days before the cleanse to avoid a strong "detox" reaction such as headaches or sluggishness. As with any cleanse, your body is eliminating the bad stuff. For some, that might manifest as mild headaches, a dip in energy, temporary changes in your body, or mild shakiness.

Some people think this is because of the cleanse itself, but really it's these two factors: Your body is ridding itself of toxins while you're flooding it with fiber and nutrients that it may not be accustomed to. Both can lead to mild discomfort in a traditional cleanse, but because our soups offer much gentler cleansing, we don't expect many of you to experience this kind of reaction. If you do, however, experience these symptoms, know that they are normally temporary. It's your body's reaction to being flooded with existing toxins from your cell tissues combined with your not giving your body the foods it's used to having (especially processed sugar—which your body learns to crave like a drug). Have some green tea or a third of a cup of coffee (black or with Almond Milk—recipe on page 148) to help your body wean off of and steer clear of overly salty or sweet foods until you reach equilibrium.

Soon enough, as your cells start functioning better, you'll feel a surge in energy—and this time it will be real, pure energy that your body is creating.

Some people report feeling more bloated after their first day on the cleanse. This is usually because they're not used to eating a lot of fiber or their bodies are not metabolizing food properly and need this reset. If this is your experience, your body will eventually figure out what to do with all the roughage goodness, and will also more readily absorb the food you give it. In the meantime, make sure to drink plenty of water. You burger and fry lovers may need five days before you feel really great, but hang in there; it will pass. And you'll feel incredible once it does!

Overall, most of our customers say that our unique cleansing program allows for a much smoother, more sensible, and totally satisfying experience. The balanced nutritional profile of the soups helps keep your metabolism and blood sugar steady, which should help to diminish any side effects of cleansing.

WHEN WILL I SEE OR FEEL RESULTS?

This of course varies for each person, but it could be as quickly as a couple of days. With the body detoxifying and receiving clean food loaded with antioxidants and phytonutrients, the shift can happen pretty quickly.

GEARING UP FOR YOUR CLEANSE

After reading about all the amazing benefits of soups and cleansing, we're sure you're ready to jump right in. But there are a few things you need to do first to ensure that your cleanse experience is as positive and beneficial as possible. You need to start shifting your diet over the course of several days so that your body can start the healing process *before* the cleanse begins. This will guarantee that it can receive all the nutrients you give it and also make sure you don't feel any of the physical discomfort that can result from shocking the system too abruptly. You'll also need to start thinking about your menus for the cleanse program you choose and start stocking your refrigerator with all the soups you need.

PREPARING THE BODY FOR CLEANSING

As we mentioned earlier, we recommend—and common sense dictates—that substances generally known to be harder on the body be eliminated two to three days before you begin cleansing. This includes foods and beverages containing caffeine, alcohol, dairy, heavy meats, refined sugars (including soda and candy), artificial chemicals, and processed foods. Ideally, you don't want to jolt your body by going cold turkey off some of your more naughty indulgences. So maybe skip that extra cup of coffee or glass of wine, and pass on that cheeseburger. Again, feel free to use green tea as a support as you wean yourself off coffee.

We've found that the best plan for transitioning to our cleanses is to replace a meal with one of our soups in the few days prior to your cleanse. This provides the body with an introduction to the high-quality healthfulness of the soups, and helps your mind align good health with a highly enjoyable, ultra-positive experience. We think it simply gets your mental attitude in the right place, which is a key factor for cleansing success. The body loves when the mind is in agreement.

You may also choose to start transitioning to a more gentle exercise regimen—maybe swapping that spin class for yoga or Pilates. While it's not necessary to wind down exercise during a soup cleanse, it is very important to listen to your own body—some bodies enjoy having a more gentle cleanse experience, while others are fine with more! We'll talk more about cleansing and exercise in chapters 7 and 8.

PREPARING THE KITCHEN
FOR CLEANSING

The beautiful thing about our soup cleanse is that you don't need to go out and buy much more than fresh ingredients. But you'll want to get your kitchen ready to receive all the nutritious bounty that's going to nourish you during your cleanse. Here's what you need:

- **Blender or food processor.** Angela loves her Vitamix, while Vivienne swears by her high-speed blender. There's no need to shell out for a fancy piece of equipment if you don't have one.
- **Standard kitchen equipment.** None of our recipes call for complicated techniques or tools, but we do recommend having a good knife for chopping fruits and vegetables, a cutting board, a couple of bowls for mixing and soaking, a baking sheet or two, a sauté pan, and of course a large soup pot.
- **Nut milk bag.** The one slightly funky item we also recommend is a nut milk bag. These are great not only for straining nut milks but also for soaking seeds, nuts, and legumes for sprouting. If you can't find one at your grocery store, we love the one from the Truly Organic Foods website. Or you can use a gallon-size paint strainer bag from a hardware store. Just be sure to give it a thorough cleaning before using it.
- **Food storage.** You'll be preparing sizable batches of soup to store in the fridge or freezer, especially the broths, so it's a good idea to invest in good-quality food storage containers. We prefer to use glass rather than plastic whenever possible and found that the Weck Tulip 91.3-ounce canning jars fit a recipe batch of soup beautifully. If you plan to freeze your soups, make sure your containers are freezer-safe.
- **Thermoses or mason jars.** When we created our soups, we wanted first and foremost for them to be portable. We also intended for most of them to be sipped, not eaten with a spoon (though of course you can do so if you prefer). We sell the Soupure soups in 12- and 16-ounce glass bottles, but you could easily substitute mason jars of the same size or a thermos. You'll want to make sure that your vessel has a spout that will accommodate a thick puree (which can clog a regular travel coffee

mug spout) and also fits in the cup holder of your car, if applicable. We also recommend that you opt for thermoses made of stainless steel versus plastic. Drink our cold soups right out of the bottle or use a straw! Just shake and drink, because we have no artificial stabilizers, so shake it up, baby!

- **Groceries.** After you figure out your cleanse menu, head to your grocery store or farmers' market and stock up, buying the best possible ingredients you can find or afford. You'll want to give yourself plenty of time to prepare the soups, especially the first time around, but not too far in advance, as soups lose nutritional integrity the longer they sit in the fridge. We love designating one day a week a "cook day" and just cranking out a bunch of recipes. If you make your soups on the Sunday before the week your cleanse begins, you'll have the freshest soups possible. Note that a good chicken broth takes at least three hours and a good vegetable broth requires about seventy-five

---

Glass versus Plastic

We have chosen food-safe, BPA-free plastic bottles to package our soups at Soupure. While we are glass lovers, sending glass to our nationwide customers can be dangerous because of potential glass breakage. At home, opt for glass whenever possible. This is because some plastic containers include substances such as polybrominated diphenyl ethers, or PBDEs (which cause reproductive problems), phthalates (another group of reproductive toxins), and bisphenol A, or BPA (which mimics estrogen in our bodies and can impair brain development as well as increase the risk for brain cancer, prostate cancer, decreased fertility, early puberty, neurological problems, and immunological changes).[1] When using plastic, select "BPA-free" options. However, avoid putting even these bottles in the microwave or dishwasher, as emerging research suggests that no plastic is safe from toxic leaching when it is heated or used to store hot liquid.[2]

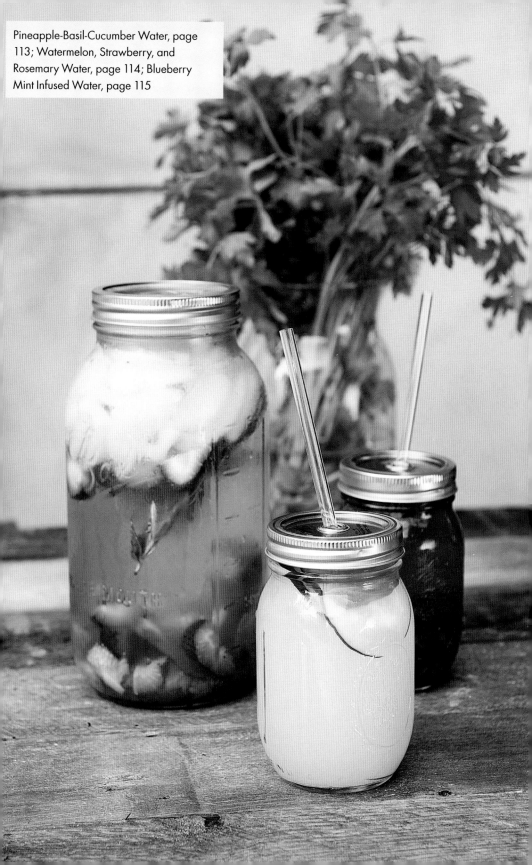

Pineapple-Basil-Cucumber Water, page 113; Watermelon, Strawberry, and Rosemary Water, page 114; Blueberry Mint Infused Water, page 115

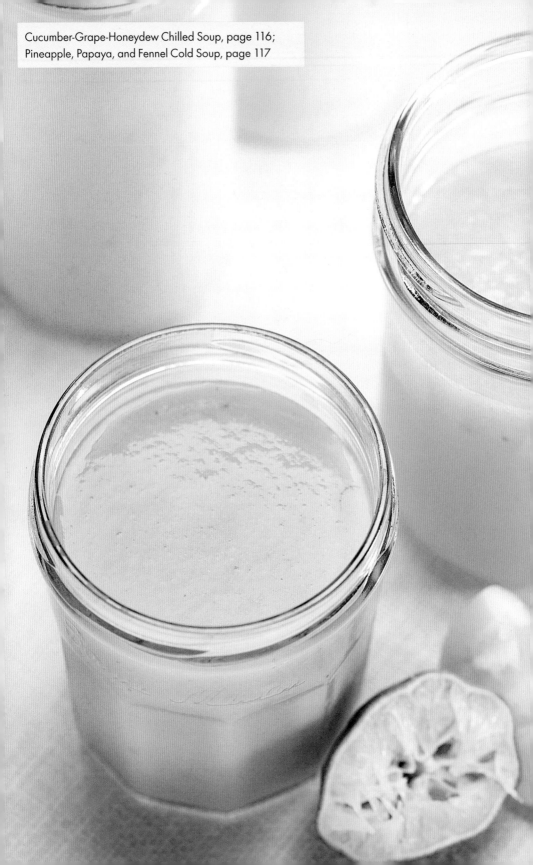

Cucumber-Grape-Honeydew Chilled Soup, page 116;
Pineapple, Papaya, and Fennel Cold Soup, page 117

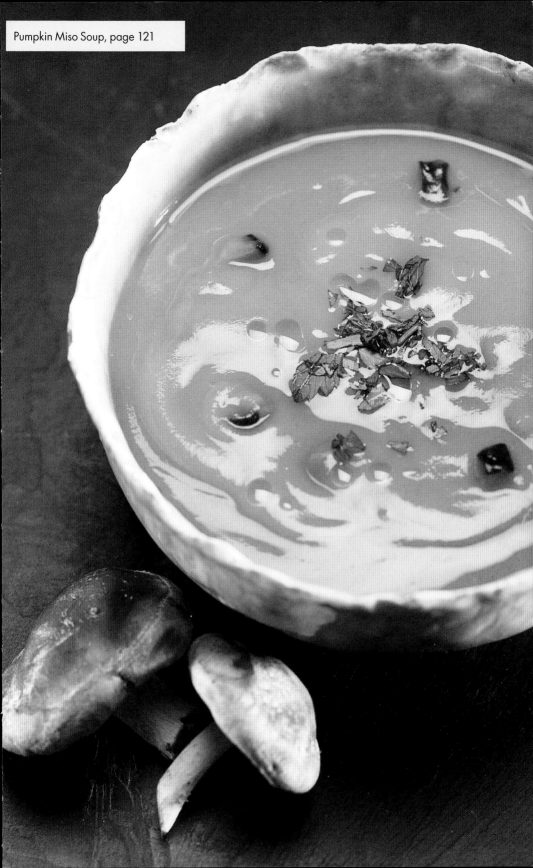

Pumpkin Miso Soup, page 121

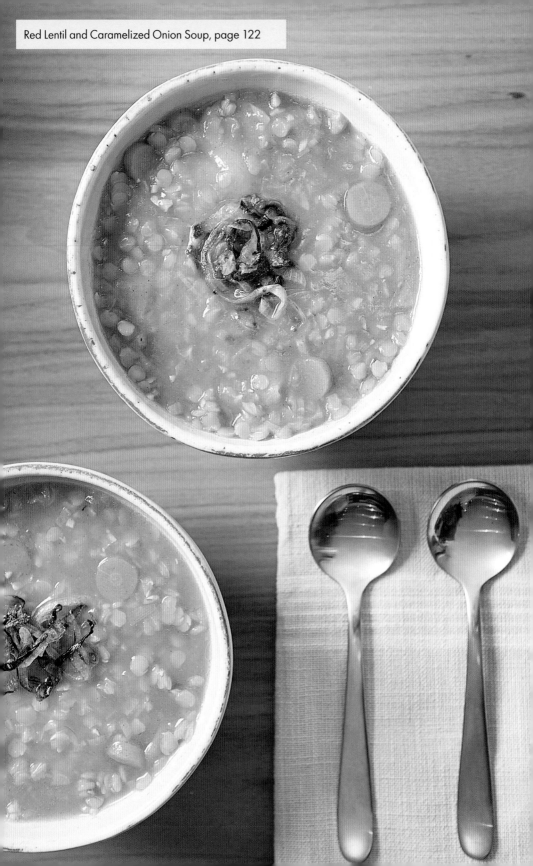

Red Lentil and Caramelized Onion Soup, page 122

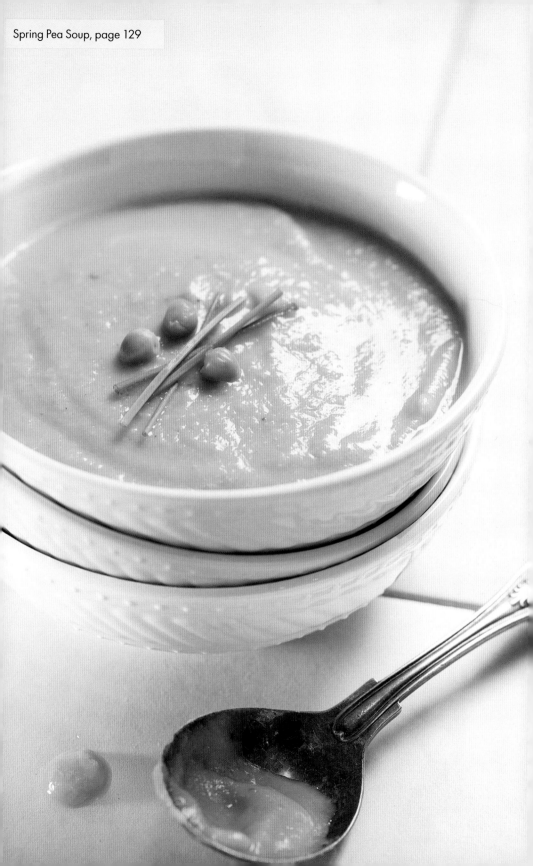

Spring Pea Soup, page 129

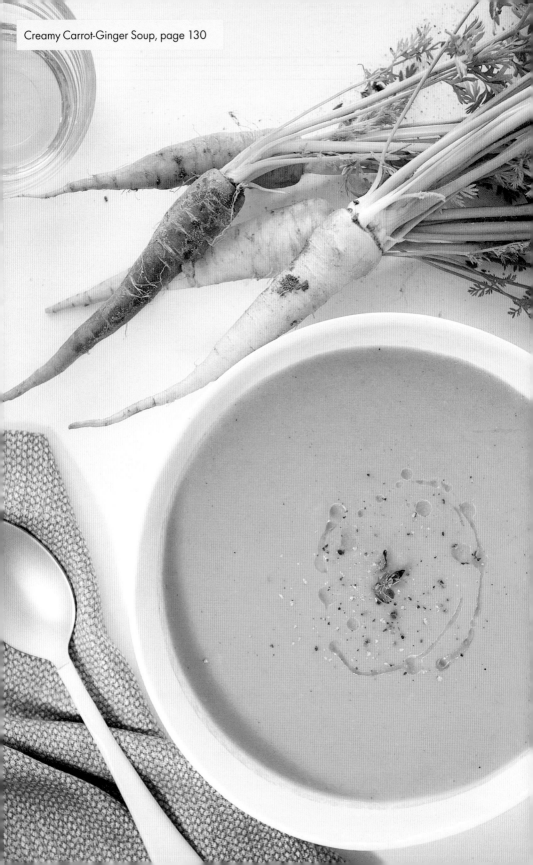

Creamy Carrot-Ginger Soup, page 130

Cauliflower Lemongrass
Soup, page 138

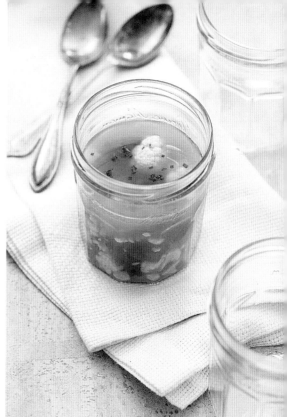

Chicken Broth, page 141

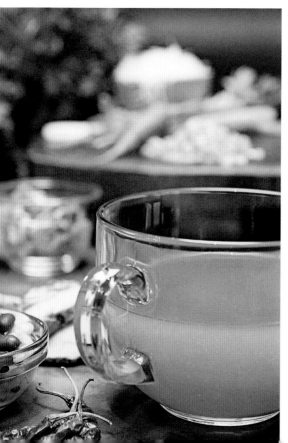

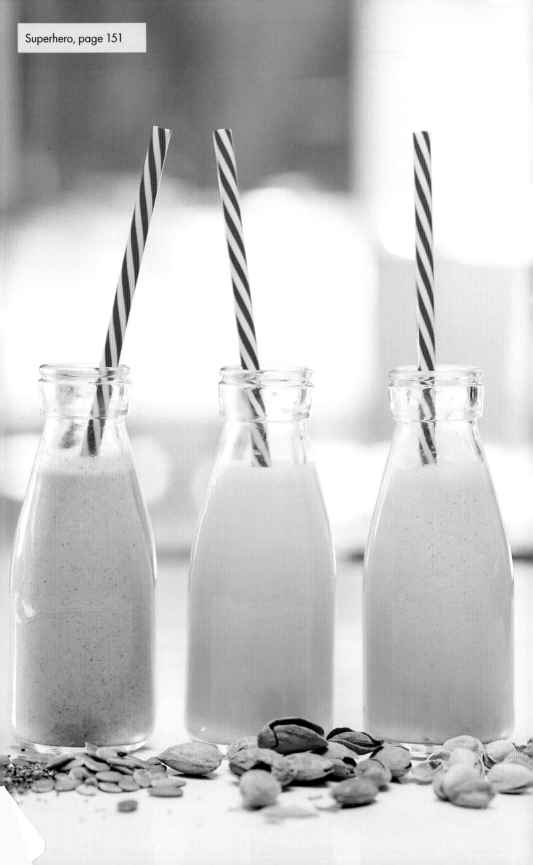

Superhero, page 151

minutes. We suggest you make loads of both and store them in the refrigerator and/or freezer so you always have them.

LET'S DO IT

You now know which program is right for you. The next chapter will give you the tools and know-how to embark on a successful cleanse journey.

I was pre-Type 2 diabetic before I started integrating Soupure into my diet. Since then, my blood sugar has totally normalized and my general health is greatly improved. The cherry on top is that all of Soupure's products are absolutely delicious and thoroughly satisfying. I'm a true believer, that's why I became a partner.

—Michael C.

7

Cleanse Menus and Instructions

As you prepare to cleanse, you'll want to start building your soup menu. Here's how we suggest structuring your days so that you're receiving everything you need in a way that benefits the body.

BUILDING YOUR CLEANSE

Ideally, enjoy each soup every couple of hours in the recommended order. Don't just gulp them down. "Chew the texture" in the soups and savor the wholeness of the ingredients we pack fresh into each bottle. A few other things to note:

- Hungry cleansers can always add a handful of almonds, celery sticks, cucumbers, or one of the snacks from our munchies list on pages 183–187.

- Active cleansers or cleansers who feel they need more fuel can add an extra Superhero (page 151), chilled or hot soup, or snacks from the munchies list.
- Go for variety. We've built this into our soup menus, but it bears repeating: You reap the most benefits from your food when you're consuming a wide variety of nutrients. If you're doing a three- or five-day cleanse, try not to eat the same soups every day. That is why our three-day cleanse offers so much variety—so you can consume over a hundred ingredients! We also recommend alternating days between having a chilled fruit-based soup and either a broth or a vegetable-based chilled soup. Too much sugar even from fruit can be bad.

ONE-DAY CLEANSE

1. **Morning starter (16 ounces) (upon awakening):** Choose from a glass of water with lemon or any of the infused waters on pages 112–115.
2. **Hot morning chaser (12 ounces) (following your starter):** Choose a broth from the section on pages 140–146.
3. **Morning nut milks or smoothies or smoothie alternatives (12 ounces) (mid-morning or post-workout):** Recipes on pages 147–152.
4. **Hot lunch soup:** Choose any of the cleanse-friendly hot soups (in the portions noted) in the section on pages 120–140.
5. **Chilled afternoon snack soup (in the portions noted):** Choose one cold soup from the section on pages 115–120.
6. **Hot dinner soup (in the portions noted):** Choose a second hot soup from the section on pages 120–140.
7. **Nightcap (in the portions noted):** Have an optional mug of broth, warmed nut milk, or latte (page 154), or Lemon-Ginger Tea (page 155).

Hydrate and Snack (optional)

- Infused water or herbal or decaffeinated tea (unlimited, all day).
- Snacks (pages 183–187) (try to limit to no more than one per day).

THREE-DAY CLEANSE

Follow instructions for the one-day cleanse for three consecutive days, but try to select at least a different hot soup or Classic Gazpacho (page 118) for lunch, a different chilled afternoon snack, and a different hot dinner soup each day.

THREE-DAY MINI-CLEANSE

Follow this schedule for three consecutive days, switching out the hot lunch soup, afternoon snack, and hot dinner soup each day.

1. **Morning starter (16 ounces) (upon awakening):** Choose from a glass of water with lemon or any of the infused waters on pages 112–115.
2. **Hot morning chaser (12 ounces) (following your starter):** Choose a broth from the section on pages 140–146.
3. **Morning nut milks or smoothies (12 ounces) (mid-morning or post-workout):** See the recipes on pages 147–152.
4. **Hot lunch soup (in the portions noted) or healthy meal substitute:** Choose any of the hot soups from the section on pages 120–140 or see the "Healthy Meal Substitutes" note on page 77.
5. **Afternoon snack soup (in the portions noted):** Choose one cold soup from the section on pages 115–120 or a broth from pages 140–146.
6. **Hot dinner soup (in the portions noted) or healthy meal substitute:** If you had a meal substitute for lunch, choose a hot soup from the section on pages 120–140. Otherwise, see the "Healthy Meal Substitutes" note on page 77.
7. **Nightcap (in the portions noted):** Have an optional mug of Lemon-Ginger Tea (page 155) or other herbal tea.

Hydrate and Snack (optional)

- Infused water or herbal or decaffeinated tea (unlimited, all day).
- Snacks (pages 183–187) (try to limit to no more than one per day).

Healthy Meal Substitutes

For your one non-soup meal a day, choose a balanced dish that's composed primarily of vegetables with protein (animal or vegetable) and
starch or whole grains. While we don't advocate eating whole animal
proteins (including muscle and fat) during our core soup cleanses, we
are all about balance. So if you're dipping your toe into the water with
a mini-cleanse and aren't ready to go cold turkey off animal protein,
it's okay to keep it in your meal rotation. We've included some recipes
to help inspire you in chapter 11, such as Sesame Garlic Chicken
and Broccoli Stir-Fry over Brown Rice (page 180) and Grilled Lemon
Chicken Salad with Market Greens and Cherry Tomatoes (page 177),
but you are also free to make up your own.

FIVE-DAY CLEANSE

Follow the one-day cleanse (page 75) for five consecutive days, but try
to have a different hot soup or Classic Gazpacho (page 118) for lunch, a
chilled afternoon snack, and a hot dinner soup at least every other day.

For Extra Credit

Kelsey De Gracia, our self-taught healing guru, likes adding two super-
boosters to his morning hydration routine: a tablespoon of apple cider
vinegar and a tablespoon of aloe vera to a glass of filtered or alkaline water. Apple cider vinegar is antibacterial and anti-inflammatory;
it regulates digestion, increases oxygenation, promotes healthy hair,
normalizes blood glucose levels, balances hormones, curbs cravings
and appetite, and maintains healthy cholesterol and circulation. Aloe
vera cleanses the digestive system, promotes weight loss, strengthens
teeth and gums, and acts as a natural laxative. As a morning elixir,
the two help further alkalize the system and soothe the digestive tract.

HOW MANY CALORIES WILL I BE CONSUMING EACH DAY?

Doctors recommend that every person should consume a minimum of 1,200 calories per day, even if dieting to the extreme. Our regular cleanses offer approximately 1,200 to 1,400 calories each day, depending on the soups or, in the case of the mini-cleanse, the meal you substitute. We make sure you get all the fiber and protein you need while not slowing you down or messing up your metabolism. We are counting for you (which is why we include portion sizes in our recipes), so don't worry about tallying the numbers—especially because we discourage traditional calorie counting as a "punishment and reward" system and encourage being mindful of your body's response to the joys of real food. There are no empty calories or nutritional tricks here, so your body will have a use for everything the soups provide.

The right amount of fuel for you depends on your body weight, activity level, and your goal for a cleanse. If you feel as though you may need more fuel, or are used to consuming a lot more calories a day and want to gently ease into having less, you may want to add soups or snacks to your cleanse. Remember, it is all about balance and what is right for you, so it is okay to supplement as long as it is healthy. More specifics on this below.

CAN I SWITCH UP THE MENU ACCORDING TO MY OWN PREFERENCE?

Of course. We recommend that you follow our order the first time around to establish a baseline. However, feel free to tailor it to your individual wants and needs. Your body will still reap the benefits from these soups, no matter the order in which they're consumed. If you are omitting a soup from the day, be sure to compensate for that nutrition. Have a handful of almonds and some dried fruit to replace one of the snack soups, or have a small salad if replacing a meal soup. When having salad, watch out for sugar-filled dressings.

WHAT IF I HAVE DIETARY RESTRICTIONS OR FOLLOW A SPECIAL DIET?

We've taken care not to add the most allergenic components to our soups, including dairy, gluten, and soy (though some broths contain miso because of its healing powers). That said, some soups do contain nuts, which you can easily replace with non-nut milks such as hemp or oat. Other considerations might include:

- **Vegan or vegetarian.** If you do not eat any animal products, simply replace our bone broths with Roasted Vegetable Broth (page 143). All our other soups are vegan, or in some cases can be made vegan by substituting honey with a vegan-friendly sweetener like coconut syrup or agave.
- **Paleo.** The Paleo principle dictates that one eat according to our caveman ancestors' traditions. This calls for a diet that includes lean meats, nuts, and berries, but excludes grains, legumes, dairy, and processed foods. All of our soups are of course free of processed products, and are also dairy-free. While some of our soups contain grains and legumes, they can be swapped out for our vegetable-based soups. In chapter 10, we've noted which of our soups are Paleo-friendly.
- **Raw.** As we mentioned earlier, we believe that some foods are best cooked in order to reap their optimal health benefits. That said, we're a big fan of plants, as are you, so let's work

something out. We've included a number of soups that have been minimally cooked (not above 115°F—if at all) and would qualify as raw. We've noted them as such in our recipe section.

MUST I CONSUME ALL SOUPS AND WATERS EACH DAY?

No, but we have carefully designed these cleanses with our nutritionist to give you all the sustenance and energy that a body needs in a day. If you don't consume all the soups or drink enough water, you may not get all the nourishment you need to be healthy. This could cause you to feel poorly or create symptoms such as headaches, dizziness, or weakness. So if you're going to skip one of our waters or soups, we encourage you to substitute something equally hydrating or nutrient-rich in its place.

That said, we believe that part of having a healthy lifestyle is getting in touch with your own mind and body. This includes knowing when you're hungry or thirsty, and when your body is fully sated. Plus, everybody is different on a different day. We've done three-day cleanses where one day we're ravenous by midafternoon, and the next we can barely finish all the soups. This can depend on your specific nutrition from the previous week, how much sleep you're getting, how active you are, and so on. Listen to your body and use common sense. If you can barely slug down your afternoon snack or your last soup of the day because you're feeling full, don't force it. Just save what you can't finish and perhaps use it later in the day when you are hungry or to supplement a day when you're feeling hungrier. If your stomach is growling or you're feeling tired and weak and want something more, it's okay to add one of our healthy snacks or a salad or a piece of fish. Balance is key. Listen to your body. If you are feeling amazing and want to turn a one-day cleanse into a two- or three-day, that's okay too!

ADDING SNACKS AND
ADDITIONAL SOUPS

As we've said before, we're not big fans of suffering for health. If your body is telling you that you need a little more food to feel supported, then don't deny it! When that happens to us, we usually reach for quick and easy options like raw veggies such as celery, cucumbers, or bell peppers, or maybe a handful of raw or roasted (but not salted or sugar-coated) nuts such as almonds, cashews, or hazelnuts. Check out pages 183–187 for a full list of our recommended snacks, both for during the cleanse and after. If you're going to be physically active during the cleanse, consider adding an additional Superhero smoothie (page 151), which will give you an energy boost that will sustain you and help your body recover more quickly with its fiber and nutrients.

WHAT TO CUT OUT DURING
YOUR CLEANSE

If you're going to go to all this trouble of cleaning out your system, then the last thing you want to do is muck it all up with things like processed foods, refined sugars, heavy fats and meats, alcohol, or caffeine. We recommend abstaining from "food crutches" like chewing gum, soda, sugary juices, caffeine, cigarettes, drugs, and alcoholic beverages in order to enhance your experience.

However, extreme lifestyle shifts should be exercised with caution. If you feel ill or unduly strained through your day, simply aim to reduce these conventional habits in a reasonable manner. Maybe aim for a third of or half a cup of coffee instead of a whole cup, or substitute green tea. We encourage you to remain aware of your progress and individual body cues.

WHAT IF I HAVE CRAVINGS DURING MY CLEANSE?

During your cleanse—and during your regular life—be mindful that cravings are information that can help you get to the bottom of what your body is asking for. Tune in to them and listen. A hankering for chocolate could be a cry for magnesium (pure cacao is loaded with the stuff). A taste for strawberries could be a request for more vitamin C. If you're craving a lot of sugar, are your blood sugar levels off? Are your cells not getting the nourishment they need, so they're looking for a new source of glucose? Are you perhaps trying to ignore certain emotions or feelings that are coming up, and eating sugar is your way of suppressing them? The body is pretty smart; we just forget to listen! Over time, though, you'll notice that eating a diet full of whole, clean foods will alleviate most, if not all, of your cravings.

REHEATING THE SOUPS: A WORD ON MICROWAVING

We each grew up using a microwave, so we completely understand their value (especially as busy professionals and mothers of three each). But now we try to shy away from relying on the microwave as the primary method for reheating our soups. Studies have shown that microwaving food can change its chemical structure, doing who-knows-what to what was once nutritionally superior soup. Heating a soup for a minute or two won't do too much pervasive damage, so it's okay in a pinch. But we don't recommend using a microwave as a primary cooking tool or means of heating your soups. And if you are going to use a microwave, steer clear of plastic containers, as their carcinogenic toxins can leach out into your food when microwaved.

BEFORE YOU BEGIN: WHAT'S YOUR "WHY?"

Our nutritionist, Marlyn, says that taking back the power of your health starts with figuring out your "why?" Why do you want to do a cleanse? Why do you want to feel better? Why do you want to lose the weight? Maybe you have that reunion or your son's big event—but what about the big picture? Do you want to live to see your kids get married and have grandkids? Do you want to be able to play with them on the floor and run around after them at the park? Maybe you want to create a business that's thriving or check things off of your life list? Or have more peaceful emotions instead of moodiness and anger? Sometimes it takes a hardship for people to connect with their why—to beat cancer or heart disease, to no longer be in pain, to live—but ideally you'd be proactive and make positive changes before it gets to that point. You have the chance to change something *now*.

Change can be overwhelming, even for those of us who have been on this path for a long time. But building health is a step-by-step approach. You can start with one baby step at a time, one action step at a time. And eventually those steps turn into a journey. Establishing and connecting with your why is your first step toward a healthier, more beautiful tomorrow and a powerful reminder of where this all began.

8

Cleansing Support: Moving, Breathing, and Sleeping

Even though it's food that's at the center of our cleanses, your body needs nourishment other than what you're eating. That's where moving, breathing, and sleeping come in. Exercise is essential for detoxification and optimal health—it moves the blood, keeps lymphatic fluid circulating, and boosts your mood. Breath is a direct connection that we have to all the physical functions that keep us balanced, happy, and calm. And sleep—*quality* sleep—is the difference between feeling run-down and depleted versus vibrant and alive. All three of these things work together to keep our systems at their strongest, namely by allowing our parasympathetic nervous system to turn on.

Our nervous system is made up of two parts: the autonomic nervous system (ANS) and the parasympathetic nervous system (PNS). You're probably more familiar with the ANS, since that's what governs our fight-or-flight response—that adrenaline-spiking response we get when we feel threatened. It's the PNS that comes in when the dust settles, to "rest and digest," or calm our bodies and return them to a more peaceful, relaxed state (something that also happens at night, but only if we're getting good-quality sleep—more on this in a bit). However, most of us are walking around in a high-stress state, meaning our ANS is *always* on high alert. When that happens, your blood pressure increases, your energy stores deplete, and your digestive function slows. Nature didn't intend for us to spend most of our lives walking around like this, and it's why so many of us are run-down, burned out, and not reaping all the nutritional benefits from the food we eat.

To alleviate this stress on our bodies, we need to activate the parasympathetic nervous system. Doing so allows your blood pressure to decrease, your pulse rate to slow, your digestion to intensify, your metabolism to rev up, and, most important, your body to heal.

While people use our cleanses in many different ways—whether it's to reset their health, heal their gut, strengthen their bones, prevent injury, or lose weight—the thing that everyone has in common is what lies at the foundation of cleansing: resetting your intentions. Maybe it starts with your diet, paying more attention to what you want to put in your temple. Or maybe it's your disposition, or clearing your mind and finding some space for a little more introspection. We're not saying you have to go into full-on Buddha mode during your cleanse, but we do believe that if you can slow down and find a little quiet during your experience, you'll see that you can do it for the rest of your life.

MOVING

Our bodies were designed to move! Movement is a part of health.

Why: It helps balance insulin levels by getting glucose moving in and out of the cells; it stimulates our telomeres—parts of our cells that affect how they age—which help slow the aging process; and it gets things moving—our blood, oxygen, our bowels. It's also one of the only ways to get the lymphatic system draining properly, which is essential for detoxification. Think of it this way: Your heart is a pump. It circulates blood throughout the body, and when blood is moving, it's pulling out toxins from the body, moving around oxygen, and basically supporting the entire ecosystem of the body. But the lymphatic system, which is responsible for filtration and cell waste cleanup, has no pump, and you have more lymphatic fluid in your body than you have blood. So if you don't move, it stagnates, junk and all. Think of a rushing waterfall with clear, blue water, and think of a pond that's been sitting stagnant and scummy in the August heat. Which would you rather drink from?

The American Cancer Society has published that exercise is one of the most powerful cancer-fighting tools. Other benefits of exercise can include lower blood pressure and a more positive outlook. Further, the National Cancer Institute reports that obesity raises the risk for many types of cancers, including cancers of the esophagus, pancreas, colon, kidney, thyroid, and gallbladder.[1] Exercising is a way of moving that fluid through your body, helping to prevent disease, while boosting oxygenation of your blood. If you're sweating, you're detoxifying.[2]

How: If you're thriving and healthy, find activities you like and mix them up—spinning, running, walking, resistance training, yoga, Pilates. We have found that the healthiest balance to aim for is an hour of cardio three to four days a week in addition to toning and stretching. During a cleanse—depending on how we're feeling—we'll either maintain our regular regimen or scale it back. Maybe we'll go 80 percent or even 50 percent in our cardio barre class versus 100 percent. The important thing to remember is that whatever you do, it is okay! Just listen to your body. You want to be mindful of not overdoing it, during a cleanse or otherwise, because that creates too much of an acidic environment in your body, which leads to inflammation. It also raises your cortisol levels, which impedes fat burning and interferes with good health.[3] Exercise should build, not deplete.

If incorporating exercise into your life is new to you, don't be afraid to start small. Commit to ten minutes of warming up three times a week, or walking for just five minutes. We're pretty sure those five minutes will stretch into thirty once you get outside and moving! Building habits takes time, but it's all about those baby steps. Remember that it's not all or nothing, and that balance is the key to sustainable, long-term health. Just remember that health and weight loss are almost entirely owing to what you put in your body. So while a movement practice is critical, it won't get you very far if you're not pairing it with eating well.

Soup Gets It Done

Traditional cleanses generally do not offer the ample amounts of protein and carbs the body needs for tissue repair after exercise. But we're not offering the typical cleanse. We hear from many of our clients that our unique blend of nutrients (including plenty of essential protein and carbohydrates) helps them maintain their active lifestyle during their detox.

BREATHING

We know what you're thinking: Don't we breathe all of the time? Of course we do, but here we're talking about the benefits of a regular breathing practice.

Why: The benefits of breathing are similar to those of exercising: It boosts circulation, increases oxygenation of the blood, regenerates cells, detoxifies the body, and turns on the parasympathetic nervous system without creating acid in the body. When that happens, you're slowing your systems down so your body uses less energy, and you're creating a perpetual calm and healing state. Breathing might seem like an easy undertaking—we do, after all, do it automatically—but most of us aren't taking the kind of deep, relaxing, and cleansing breaths that the body needs to trigger these functions. Watch a small child—see how deeply they're breathing from their belly? Over time, we forget how to breathe like that. As a result, we lose our connection to our bodies and our breath and get stuck inside our minds.

How: Having a breathing practice doesn't mean sitting in the lotus position for an hour. It can be as simple as taking deep breaths through your nose. I recommend associating breath with things you do every day—taking a shower, getting in the car, even going to the bathroom. Then use that time as a reminder to take five big breaths. Don't force it or hold it, just let it flow from your belly. Another option is to set aside just five minutes in the morning and/or evening to do nothing but sit or lie still and breathe. No to-do lists, no mentally redecorating the living room, just being present and quiet.

If you make breathing a habit, then you'll be more aware of your breath in general—whether you're holding it or your stomach is tight (which can cause stagnation in your system). If you are stressed and tight, an easy trick is to sigh or yawn. These are two of the quickest ways that your body destresses and puts itself back into a state of homeostasis. Neuroscience shows that even dogs yawn when they have anxiety and that fish will yawn before making a decision.[4] Pretty amazing!

From the Self-Taught Healer and Our Health Geek: Kelsey De Gracia

My introduction to health—though I didn't know it at the time—was through my Japanese grandmother. Unbeknownst to her, she was always teaching me about basic traditional types of Japanese food, which have a symbiotic relationship with the body. When she was ninety-three, I decided to put those remedies to use and become her full-time caretaker. I wanted to find ways to help her rebuild her body, so she could stay independent for as long as possible.

My focus became combining traditional Japanese eating with a Western regenerative diet, healing on the cellular level, and stimulating the cells and organs in order to rejuvenate the body. I started reading about food medicine and traditional methods of eating and healing. I knew I was on the right track when I was traveling in France and found a book from medieval Europe that was very similar to books from traditional Chinese medicine.

For my grandmother, I was combining diet, exercise, and also a breathing regimen, in addition to intuitive touch therapy like chi quong. I believed it was stimulating her body on a deeper level than anything else could. Over time, I was able to restore her right arm's full range of motion, which had been severely limited, get her walking comfortably again, and ultimately return her to the golf course and garden, where she spent her time until she died at ninety-seven. Seeing this amazing transformation—she could walk better at ninety-seven than she did at ninety!—and witnessing what was possible was my "Oh my God" moment. I called upon these same methods when I had my own health challenges, and again when my dog was diagnosed with skin cancer and given one year to live (she's still alive, eight years later). I believe wholeheartedly that it was a nourishing diet combined with a gentle movement practice and breathing techniques that gave my family the gift of health as well as love and laughter.

SLEEPING

Nourishing the body also includes proper rest. It's a huge part of the wellness equation because the body needs rest to repair and rejuvenate.

Why: Good-quality sleep allows the parasympathetic nervous system to turn on, calm the body's systems, and tend to all necessary maintenance. This means a good, long stretch of restful sleep, about seven to eight hours.

How: Being mindful of the circadian rhythms dictated by nature will help you get the best, deepest sleep possible. Ideally you'd go to bed in the 10 p.m. hour and wake up seven to eight hours later. Make sure your bedroom is dark, because any light coming in can trigger the body to think it's daylight, so it might not produce as much melatonin (a hormone that helps regulate sleep and waking cycles). And be sure to remove any stress-provoking items in the room like a computer.

If you need help relaxing at the end of the day, essential oils can be nice—especially lavender. And sometimes food can help support good sleep by balancing your blood sugar in the evening. Some warmed nut milk (pages 147–152) or a spoonful of almond butter is an easy-to-digest remedy. Exercise also supports healthy sleep, as does hydration. You can also try doing a "brain dump" before bed, or writing down all the thoughts in your head so you can clear your mind for sleep. Above all, remember that health supports health. So if you're eating healthfully all day, getting movement, and handling the stressful elements of your life, your sleep will be better.

Keep a Detox Journal

Writing in a journal is a great way to slow down and be more aware of how your body is responding to the cleanse. Jot down how you're feeling physically to see if you can fine-tune your diet even more specifically to your needs. If you notice that you're feeling great until about 3 or 4 p.m., when all of a sudden you're exhausted, then that's a time when you need a little more support. Maybe it's green tea for a little caffeine or a little healthy protein from some nuts. This is a great way to start becoming aware of the energy-related rhythms of your day and also noticing the cause and effect of what you're eating.

Journaling is also a wonderful emotional outlet. Have any feelings come up since you started the cleanse? Do you think the way you used to eat might have been because of certain things in your life you haven't wanted to sort out?

Or maybe sitting for a few moments with a blank page and a pretty pen can be another opportunity to connect with your intentions and goals for the new and improved you.

DETOX WORKSHEET

We created this fun little worksheet to help you take inventory of the amazing changes you'll see while cleansing. Before you begin your cleanse, check all the boxes in the "before" column that apply to your current state of health. As you go through the process, begin checking the "after" boxes that apply—and crossing off the ones that don't any longer!

Before

☐ Acne
☐ Allergies
☐ Anxiety
☐ Bad breath
☐ Bloating
☐ Brain fog
☐ Constipation
☐ Depression
☐ Digestive problems
☐ Eczema
☐ Fatigue
☐ Food cravings
☐ Foul-smelling stools

☐ Gas
☐ Headaches
☐ Heartburn
☐ Joint pain
☐ Low energy
☐ Low sex drive
☐ Muscle aches
☐ Puffy eyes or dark circles
☐ Sinus issues
☐ Skin rashes
☐ Sleep problems
☐ Water retention
☐ Weight challenges

After

- ☐ Better breath
- ☐ Better mood
- ☐ Clear eyes
- ☐ Clear thinking
- ☐ Feeling "light"
- ☐ Glowing skin
- ☐ Increased comfort in body
- ☐ Improved sense of well-being
- ☐ Improved sex drive
- ☐ Less buildup on the tongue and teeth
- ☐ More energy
- ☐ Reduced or eliminated cravings
- ☐ Regular bowel movements
- ☐ Restful sleep
- ☐ Stronger hair
- ☐ Weight loss

One of the things that we love most about a soup cleanse is that the benefits don't stop with your cleanse. It's incredibly easy to incorporate the basic tenets of a soup cleanse into everyday life, which makes this program much more lifestyle-friendly than other cleanses where it's essentially feast or famine. In the next chapter, we'll give you all the tools and ideas for carrying this amazing post-cleanse feeling with you.

9

Back to (Better Than) Normal: Incorporating Soups into Everyday Life

Congratulations! You've made it through your cleanse and you're (most likely) feeling vibrant and well. Though your official detox may have come to an end, that doesn't mean you can't keep cleaning up your act. In fact, by following the advice we lay out in this chapter, you can set yourself up for optimal health all the time—not just when you're cleansing.

We recommend coming out of a cleanse the same way you went into it: gently and gradually. Choose from clean, whole plant–based foods and reduce or avoid processed, sugary foods, caffeine, and alcohol. Then gradually add in foods that are heavier and more difficult to digest, like animal foods. So, for example, if you eat meat, you might start by introducing your body to fish, then to chicken, and then to beef. This way you're not shocking your system back into its old patterns of a perpetually panicked state, while you are also creating the foundation for a lifetime of healthy eating habits. You can still have soup for lunch or dinner as you exit your cleanse. We like having soup for lunch at least three times a week to help keep our tummies flat and our bodies feeling good.

EATING FOR LIFE

One of the things we love most about souping is that it's not an abrupt departure from a normal diet. While you're being gentler on your digestive system than usual, and you're taking extra care not to take in too much sugar—healthy or otherwise—or heavier, hard-to-digest foods, you're still *eating*.

As you transition back into your "normal" diet, don't forget the lessons you learned while cleansing. Think about the rhythm of your day, how you gently woke up your body in the morning, gave it tons of fuel during the day with frequent hits of energy, and then gradually allowed it to rest for the night. You loaded up on foods that gave you all the nutrients you needed, while avoiding damaging foods. This is how you eat for life.

YOUR NEW PLATE

Now that the cleanse is over and you're transitioning back to solid foods, we recommend changing the way you think about the ratio of different foods on your plate. If you look at your plate and divide it in half, and take one half and divide it in two, that's the foundation of how you should think about your meals. Ideally, half of your dish would be filled with vegetables, one-quarter with protein (plant or animal—about the size of your palm), and another quarter with gluten-free grains or starchy vegetables.

And just because the cleanse is over doesn't mean you're done with deliciously nourishing soups! Continue working the soups into your regular diet. They taste so good and it is so easy to enjoy and include them. Make a batch to keep in your refrigerator and just grab and go. Have one every day, a few times a week, or whenever you're in the mood. They're a great way to support your health and wellness in an ongoing, sustainable way, and best of all to make you feel and look your best.

- **Vegetables**. As we said before, aim to eat the rainbow. Over the course of a week, try to get as many colors on your plate as you can. We love going to the farmers' market for inspiration, since it's easy to get into a veggie rut. Bring something new home from the market or store each trip, and before long you'll have a strong and varied rotation to choose from. By making sure to load up your plate (or bowl or mug) with veggies for most meals during the day—whether roasted, sautéed, stir-fried, pureed, or tossed in a salad—you're giving yourself an insurance policy in case you're eating too much of the not-so-great stuff.

- **Grains and starches**. Starchy vegetables and grains ultimately break down into sugar. While their fiber does help mitigate the effects of that sugar on your body, you don't want to eat an unlimited amount at each meal. Some good options for starchy vegetables include peas, parsnips, potatoes, pumpkin, squash, zucchini, corn, and yams. We recommend sticking primarily to gluten-free grains (such as brown rice, quinoa, millet, amaranth, non-wheat-contaminated oats, gluten-free noodles), but eating the occasional whole grains with gluten (barley, rye, spelt, farro, semolina) can be perfectly all right so long as your body feels good afterward (more on that in a bit).

- **Animal protein**. When it comes to eating animals and their eggs, make sure you're getting the cleanest sources: grass-fed beef; organic, cage-free chicken; and meat sourced from animals that are responsibly raised, fed a biologically appropriate (grain-free) diet, not given hormones or antibiotics, and not injected with sodium nitrate "plumpers." You won't always find this information on a label, which is why it's important to have a good relationship with the butcher or farmer who's providing these things.

Since meat can have an acidic effect on the body, consider combining it with something alkaline like greens, which will help neutralize it in the digestive system.

- **Fish.** Whenever possible, buy wild. Most farmed fish in this country—especially farm-raised salmon—are given an unnatural grain-based diet and are pumped up with antibiotics. There's such a thing as farmed fish that are "raised by the ocean," which is a little healthier. But wild is best, even if you're deciding between frozen wild and fresh farmed. Check to see which fish are in season in your area and buy extra to freeze.

- **Plant-based proteins.** These mainly include beans and lentils (though there are some grains, like quinoa, that pack a big protein punch). Note that legumes contain a protective coating that prevents them from being broken down and digested, and this can actually keep you from digesting other nutrients as well. That's why we recommend soaking them overnight and then rinsing them before cooking them. If you're using canned beans, opt for a BPA-free or Tetra Pak version, and rinse off the starches.

From Marlyn the Nutritionist: The ACE Plan

Everyone likes to ace their tests, work, projects, life—everyone likes an A. So I came up with this simple formula for remembering how to build healthy, long-lasting eating habits:

A for **Add in**
C for **Crowd out**
E for **Elevate up**

It's all about making choices and phasing out the not-so-great ones—**add in** more healthy foods to **crowd out** the unhealthy ones, and **elevate up** your old food crutches with healthier options. Even if you do nothing but add in more vegetables, you're still taking steps toward better health. Over time, as you add in more nutrient-rich foods, your cravings will shift, your body will feel better, and you'll naturally start to crowd out foods that aren't giving you that sense of wellness. You'll eventually be eating less sugar, fewer chemicals, fewer processed foods. You might still have that craving for chocolate chip cookies, but maybe you'll make your own at home with your own healthier ingredients, or you'll go to an organic bakery.

YOUR NEW DAILY RHYTHM

Just as there's an optimal way to eat the soups during a cleanse, there's an ideal way to eat throughout the day that's most beneficial for your body. It's based on wisdom gleaned from ancient practices like traditional Chinese medicine and Ayurveda. And don't forget to add in lots of hydration as you go!

- **First thing in the morning (6 a.m. to 10 a.m.).** Your digestive fire isn't fully revved yet, so this is a good time for something that's already been broken down by the blender and is easy to digest. One of our infused waters, a chilled soup, or one of our broths is a great way to start the day. You're getting plenty of nourishment without taking up a lot of the body's energy to digest.
- **Breakfast.** We like to have a little protein by 10 a.m. Whether it's a bowl of oatmeal, muesli, a Superhero smoothie (page 151), or an omelet, some protein plus a little healthy fat and fiber supports feeling satisfied and fends off cravings. See pages 156–159 for some of our favorite breakfast recipes. Add

a Japanese sweet potato to a breakfast omelet? Who knew how healthy a potato could be?

- **Morning snack.** Unless you're fasting or eating more frequently because of a specific health challenge, we recommend eating every three to four hours to support your blood sugar and keep it balanced, which in turn keeps your body balanced. At each of these intervals, your body usually needs some protein, whether vegetable or animal, to support its repairs. Otherwise it might be taking that nutrition from its own muscle mass. See pages 183–187 for our favorite quick and easy snack options.

- **Lunchtime.** This is your most important meal of the day. Think back to that mental image of your plate or bowl—loaded half-full with veggies plus a protein and a starch. Maybe it's a mug of our Beef Barley Soup (page 175), Roasted Eggplant and Lentil Soup (page 132), or Grilled Lemon Chicken Salad with Market Greens and Cherry Tomatoes (page 177).

- **Afternoon snack.** When you hit that classic afternoon energy dip, don't try to power through until dinner. So many people don't eat during the day because they're busy and running on adrenaline (and most likely caffeine). That usually means that between 4 p.m. and 9 p.m. they're making up for it. But when you eat too much energy-dense food at night, you set off a cascade of unhealthy ramifications: You usually aren't able to fall asleep at a healthy time (which messes up your natural rhythms), your body is using its energy to digest while you sleep instead of repair, and your parasympathetic nervous system can't click on, so you'll wake up feeling sluggish and tired (which usually leads to making poor food choices and the beginning of a vicious cycle). Our recommendation: Head off that midday slump with a chilled soup, a vegetable or bone broth, a chilled nut milk smoothie, or any of our suggestions on pages 183–187. If you are a coffee drinker, try one of our teas or lattes instead.

- **Dinner.** As we mentioned above, dumping a lot of food into your body right before it needs to rest leads to poor digestion, poor sleep, and wasted energy. Ease your body toward sleep with a lighter but satisfying meal. Any of our soups would be wonderful, or have a piece of fish with veggies like our Baked Wild Salmon with Avocado, Ginger, and Mango Salsa (page 179).
- **Pre-sleep treat:** Sometimes you want a little something before sleep. This is the perfect time for one of our teas or lattes (pages 153–155), or a mug of Roasted Vegetable Broth (page 143).

From Marlyn the Nutritionist:
Be Your Own Food Detective

Many times I see people come into my practice with allergies, mood swings, headaches, bloat, skin eruptions, and so on, and often these symptoms pop up in a person's life out of seemingly nowhere. What I do is ask them to think back to when they were feeling good, and then we work from there to identify what might have changed.

The next time you have a breakout/headache/sleepless night/ poor digestion, look at what might have triggered it. Whether it's diet-related, emotional, or hormonal, that's information about what might not be supporting your body. Even though a food may be "good," like a whole grain that contains gluten, it might not be for your body. You need to be your own health advocate, because you know your body best, and these discomforts are keeping you from the things you love most in life.

STORE-BOUGHT FOOD

We've included tons of our favorite recipes in this book, and we can't recommend more highly doing the cooking yourself as a path to health. While we'll talk about that in much more detail in the next chapter, we want to acknowledge that you might not be ready to jump into full kitchen-warrior mode. If you do continue buying prepared or packaged foods from the store, be sure to read the label and look for products that have five to seven ingredients at most and that are made from whole, non-GMO, preferably organic ingredients without refined sweeteners. As we mentioned before, even organic products can contain preservatives, additives, and fillers. Broths in particular can be a pitfall, since many of them contain MSG. Here is a simple rule: If you can't pronounce an ingredient, don't put it in your body!

SUGAR

As you know by now, we don't advocate eating processed sugar in any of its millions of forms—high-fructose corn syrup, palm sugar, cane sugar, dextrose, maltose, or any other form. Sugar overload is at the root of most, if not all, of our health challenges, so it's crucial that you're mindful about how much you're putting into your body and where it comes from. We recommend using natural sweeteners that are gentle on the body: dates, dried apricots, coconut sugar, raw honey, or a little bit of coconut or maple syrup.

WHAT ABOUT COFFEE?

Coffee has been used in Chinese medicine for healing purposes. It can help the metabolism and boost circulation and flow in your system, but then again, coffee is very acidic, which you know from page 13 can cause the body to be more acidic. And the more acidic your body is, the more prone to disease you are. Plus, your liver, a key detoxifying organ, needs to work hard to metabolize coffee. And coffee has a ten-hour half-life, so it stays in your blood system longer than you'd think and can impede your sleep.

So the role that coffee has in your diet comes back to balance. Are you having two cups or nine? Are you addicted? Are you drinking it because you have no energy when you should be evaluating why you're dragging instead of reaching for that extra cup of joe? Is it something that's really supporting you? If you don't think green tea with maca will be a satisfying substitute, then just be mindful of when and why you're drinking coffee. And buy the highest-grade organic coffee you can find.

IS THERE A PLACE FOR BOOZE IN MY DIET?

We're all about balance, and that includes having a good time. We've even included some really fun boozy twists on a few of our juices and infused waters in chapter 11. That said, wine, beer, and spirits break down into sugar in your body, so you do want to look at the total load of sugar you're taking in in a day. If you're going to have wine, maybe have less fruit or starchy vegetables that day. Be sure to balance drinking with healthier habits like exercising and hydrating (especially because alcohol is very dehydrating). And think about how you're using that drink—is it something to enhance your meal and relax? Or are you using it to cover up emotions or things you don't want to deal with? Has it become a habit? A dependence? As with anything else, it goes back to discipline and the big picture of creating your healthiest self. If you find that you've lost the sense of balance that you gained during your cleanse, give yourself a one-day cleanse to reboot, restore, and recalibrate.

THIS IS WHERE WE LEAVE YOU

Our sincerest congratulations on making it to the end of this part of the book—though certainly not the end of your healing journey. We hope that you'll use this book again and again, as a resource and a cheerleader. The thoughts, tips, and other wisdom we've included here are things that we consistently refresh ourselves with, so that we can continue to remember just how important it is to give our bodies all the nutrition and support they need—and how delicious and fun it can be! Remember to be patient with yourself, be kind, and don't be afraid to take it one day at a time. Now go forth and soup!

Part III

THE RECIPES

10

Core Cleanse Recipes

At Soupure, we don't approve a recipe until we know it offers you the ultimate taste experience. By looking to the best professional culinary talent and working with expert nutritional advisers, we have curated a superior collection of nourishing hot and cold soups, healing broths, hydrating infused waters, indulgent nut milks, and curative teas and lattes. The recipes in this chapter and the one that follows are as healthy for you as they are delicious. In addition to including all of the recipes you need to follow the cleanse, we've also included some of our favorites for supplementing the soups during a mini-cleanse or for enjoying in everyday life, from easy-to-grab snacks and simple veggie dishes to nutritious entrees, desserts, and even cocktails. That's right, because even soup can get a little naughty.

We've spent countless hours devoted to achieving the perfect balance of savory and sweet, layering complexity and depth of flavor, fine-tuning perfect texture, and exploring powerful and therapeutic combinations of foods—we've put in the work so you don't have to! These recipes don't require fancy gadgets or complicated techniques, just a sense of adventure and a desire to feel absolutely amazing.

Not too keen on cooking? We don't blame you. But consider this: Most store-bought prepared foods—especially from the deli or cold and hot bar—are loaded with added sugars, preservatives, and fillers. It's tricky to know exactly what that food is made from and what the ingredients truly are. Even those that start out nutrient-dense can be cooked so aggressively that all the good stuff is lost. Labels can be deceiving—sugar can come in so many forms, and ingredients that seem innocent on the label, like "natural flavors," may actually trigger health challenges. Why use your time scrolling through an impossible-to-read label when you can buy seasonal, fresh ingredients and make your own healthy creations at home? With a little planning and a bit of preparation, cooking can be a fantastic addition to a healthy lifestyle, and healthy body too!

But that doesn't mean you have to spend hours slaving away in the kitchen—far from it. Think about how you can make the work easier for yourself: Buy pre-chopped veggies or shop in the frozen section (frozen fruits and veggies are picked and frozen at the height of their freshness and haven't lost any nutrients!). Or maybe pick a day of the week on which you do nothing but wash and prep your veggies, and another day to cook, so it's more relaxing. Can you engage your partner, children, roommate, neighbor, or friends to help? Swapping a delicious home-cooked meal for some dishwashing is a pretty sweet deal.

Think about cooking for yourself and your family less as a chore and more as a treat. You *get* to make yourself the most healing, nutritious food possible. You certainly won't get all of these benefits from store-bought soups and packaged foods. You have the opportunity to make yourself delicious meals free of fillers, additives, excess salt and sugar, artificial coloring, pesticides, GMOs, and all the other junk that robs you of nutrients, damages your body, and makes you sick.

So put some music on, light a candle, pour yourself a glass of wine, and embrace the experience. Play, experiment, enjoy! Invite friends and family over for a meal and have them bring some of your favorite dishes from this book. Our kids learned a lot about measurements and following directions by helping out and having fun in the kitchen. Or set up a soup swap so you can stock your fridge or freezer with a wide array of options. Instant cleanse!

We hope you enjoy the recipes in this chapter—we've lovingly developed, tested, and tasted them with the Soupure team. These soups are straight from our kitchens to yours! Before you dig in, we want you to hear directly from one of the people who helped us come up with our Soupure product line—Joli Robinson, our head chef. Soupure's culinary vision has evolved from the collective efforts of many chefs and nutritionists, but today it is guided by Joli and Kelsey De Gracia, our head of production. Both Joli and Kelsey have drawn from their own personal struggles with food to help us create and refine products for Soupure that not only provide the fullest spectrum of nutrients, but also taste delicious.

From Our Chef:
Joli Robinson, Executive Chef of Soupure

My own plight with the damaging effects of gluten really helped wake me up to the importance of putting the right foods into your body that work for you, instead of against you. No one ever knew that my ailments as a child were a result of food sensitivities. I didn't even find out until my early twenties, so I spent the majority of my life unnecessarily suffering. I always felt like my body was working against me, even though I was doing and eating a lot of the things people considered "healthy." I was lucky enough to cross paths with a woman named Rose Marie Swift, who had her own health battles. She helped me figure out what was going on with my body and how food affected it. It turned my life around. It is hard to believe that my lethargy and feeling so bad for so long was all food-related. Discovering wellness spurred a passion to find out what else I could learn to make myself feel even better.

Three years ago, I left my job in New York and moved to California. I began working with some very talented chefs, went to culinary school, and started cooking for private clients. I not only learned the technical aspects of cooking, but also how food can nourish and support your body—while tasting delicious! I believe that clean, pure eating is the best way to be healthy and live vibrantly. If you take care of your body, it will take care of you.

I know exactly what it feels like to be burdened with a diet that is actually damaging instead of nourishing, and my heart goes out to everybody who suffers unnecessarily. My own personal path to health has taught me that you do not have to sacrifice taste for well-being. You can have the best of both worlds, and you can approach food creatively in the exact same way an artist approaches a canvas. We hope you love our soups, waters, teas, and remedies as much as we do. Cheers to our health and happiness!

HOW LONG WILL THE SOUPS STAY FRESH?

We recommend storing our soups for only three days for optimal freshness. After that, the nutritional integrity of the soup begins to decline. So if you're doing a five-day cleanse, either you'll need to prepare two batches of soups, or you can freeze a portion of one large batch (see page 109). We have a special process for fast cooling that will extend our Soupure soups for longer, so if you purchase your soups from us, you have a bit more time.

Since you will be cooling your freshly made hot soups at home, we recommend using one of these two cooling methods before you refrigerate or freeze them.

Option one: Pour your finished soup into a large glass storage container or several smaller containers (many recipes fit into a two-quart mason jar or two one-quart mason jars). Fill a large pot (a Dutch oven or pasta pot works well) with ice and place your open soup container(s) in the middle of the ice. Carefully add water to the ice to fill the pot and surround your soup. Stir every half hour so that the soup chills completely (safety standards say about 40 degrees). Seal your airtight containers with lids and place them in the refrigerator or freeze.

Option two: Fill a sink with ice. When you've finished making your soup, place the entire saucepan in the ice-filled sink. Carefully add water so that the pot is immersed, but water is not spilling in. Stir soup every half hour so that it chills completely. When soup is cooled pour it into airtight containers and place in the refrigerator or freeze.

FREEZING OUR SOUPS

A great way to prep our meals in advance—especially for a cleanse—is to batch cook then freeze our soups. They're great frozen so long as you freeze them while they're still fresh, which is right after they've cooled. While freezing in airtight containers when the product is fresh won't change the nutritional value, it can change the consistency (some soups freeze better than others). For example, a fully pureed soup will freeze well. Frozen soups with mushrooms and other vegetables can change the texture of those vegetables. We especially prefer not to freeze shiitake mushroom soup due to texture change. Once you've defrosted the soup, whisk it well while heating on the stove—and perhaps add a little water to thin it—and it should be good as new.

A WORD ON ORGANIC INGREDIENTS

These recipes call for using organic ingredients whenever possible. Refer back to pages 48–49 for the "Clean Fifteen"—foods that are suitable non-organic alternatives. If you're going to be using a piece of produce skin and all, then it's even more important to buy organic.

WATER

With the exception of our alkaline water recipes, assume that we're calling for filtered water (because alkalinity is lost when water is heated). Use the best-quality water you can. For a refresher on why this is essential, see pages 53–54.

SALT

Though our soups contain far, far less sodium than a can of store-bought soup, they do contain salt. That's because this mineral in moderation is essential for body function, especially helping the brain and nerves send electrical impulses. We just make sure to use it sparingly and also to use the best quality possible. Our recipes call for sea salt, which is produced through evaporation of ocean water or saltwater lakes, and usually has been processed minimally. As a result, it contains trace minerals like potassium, iron, and zinc and helps balance the pH levels in the body. Table salt, on the other hand, is composed of sodium chloride, which is not a form of salt that is natural to the body. It's also heavily processed to eliminate minerals and usually contains an anticaking agent to prevent clumping. As a result, it can be difficult for the body to digest. We recommend that you invest in a high-quality sea salt—it will last you for ages!

WASHING YOUR HERBS AND PRODUCE

We highly recommend washing your produce and fresh herbs before cooking. Even though organically grown food isn't grown with pesticides, it still can come into contact with fertilizers, bugs, and bacteria—which, no matter how natural they are, aren't exactly tasty ingredients. Plus, in order to get to you in the grocery store, they have to be handled by the farmer, farming equipment, grocery store employees, and most likely other shoppers. Bottom line: You just never know.

Luckily, it's easy to remove germs and bacteria (and even some pesticides) by using a store-bought produce wash or making your own. We prefer the latter since you know for a fact that there aren't any hidden chemicals. Here's a recipe we love:

1 cup water

1 cup white or cider vinegar

1 tablespoon baking soda

2 tablespoons fresh lemon juice

Optional: A couple of drops of essential oils such as lavender, grapefruit, or lemongrass

Combine the ingredients in a spray bottle, give your fruit and veggies a good spritz, let them sit for 5 minutes, then rinse.

THE KEY TO SUCCESS

All our cleanse recipes are free from dairy, refined sugar, white flour, and other processed ingredients, in addition to other high-inflammation foods. The following keys, when they appear at the top of a recipe, tell you other helpful details to know:

(L) Recommended lunch soup

(D) Recommended dinner soup

(GF) Gluten-free (but always check ingredients with your own health practitioner if you suffer from serious gluten allergies or celiac disease)

(PF)   Paleo-friendly

(V)   Vegan; (V) in parentheses denotes that there is a non-vegan
      ingredient that can be substituted or omitted

(R)   Raw

INFUSED WATERS

We get it, sometimes plain water can be, well, so unsatisfying. But juice, soda, and artificially flavored waters have all that refined sugar and other nasty additives. Plus, there's nothing that comes close to water when it comes to detox power. It helps flush out everything you don't want in the body, and supports and nourishes all the organs, tissues, and cells that keep things running smoothly. To help entice you and make it easier to add water into your routine, we add our own "spa alkaline waters," that is, alkaline-infused with fruit and herbs. Not only are they beautiful to look at, but they taste delicious and give you the hydration you need when cleansing. The flavor is subtle—don't expect something super-sweet—but they offer just enough of something tasty and fresh to make your daily hydration a treat. These waters also look so pretty poured into a glass pitcher or mason jar, making them perfect for parties. We created them to go alongside our cleanse but love them so much we drink them every day, cleansing or not. We've used one of these recipes as a base for the Blueberry Mojito (page 188). When you are not cleansing and you want to jazz up a cocktail, get creative with the infused waters!

We've included three of our favorite combinations here, but feel free to experiment. There are endless delicious mash-ups. These recipes call for using alkaline water, but filtered water works too!

Pineapple-Basil-Cucumber Water

YIELD: About 6 cups
CLEANSE SERVING SIZE: 16 ounces
PREP TIME: 12 minutes

---

2 cups skinned and cubed pineapple
6 cups alkaline water
6 basil leaves
1 small cucumber, sliced thinly
Ice

Add half of the pineapple cubes to a blender, and pour in just enough alkaline water to cover. Blend on low speed and set aside.

Place the basil in a 2-quart pitcher or mason jar and use a muddler or the handle end of a wooden spoon or spatula to gently press against the basil leaves and twist. This will slightly bruise the leaves and release their flavor—no need to smash them into bits!

Add the sliced cucumber and remaining pineapple cubes to the container and muddle as you did the basil leaves, just enough to release their juices.

Pour the contents of the blender into the pitcher or jar and stir. Top off the container with water and chill. You can drink this right away, but the flavor intensifies as it soaks, so we recommend letting it sit for a couple of hours or even overnight. Serve as-is with ice or use a fine-mesh strainer to sieve out the fruit and herb bits.

WATERMELON, STRAWBERRY, AND ROSEMARY WATER

YIELD: About 6 cups
CLEANSE SERVING SIZE: 16 ounces
PREP TIME: 10 minutes

---

1 sprig fresh rosemary
10 large strawberries, quartered
1 cup cubed watermelon
6 cups alkaline water
Ice

Place the rosemary in a 2-quart pitcher or mason jar and use a muddler or the handle end of a wooden spoon or spatula to gently press against the leaves and twist. This will slightly bruise the rosemary and release its flavor—no need to smash it into bits!

Add the strawberries and watermelon to the container and muddle as you did the rosemary, just enough to release their juices. If you'd like, leave some strawberries whole or halved for a pretty touch.

Top off the container with water. Stir again and chill. You can drink this right away, but the flavor intensifies as it soaks, so we recommend letting it sit for a couple of hours or even overnight. Serve as-is with ice or use a fine-mesh strainer to sieve out the fruit and herb bits.

BLUEBERRY MINT INFUSED WATER

YIELD: About 6 cups
CLEANSE SERVING SIZE: 16 ounces
PREP TIME: 5 minutes

2 sprigs fresh mint
1 cup organic blueberries
6 cups alkaline water
Ice

Place the mint (the whole sprig, or leaves picked so they swirl around in the water) in a 2-quart pitcher or mason jar and use a muddler or the handle end of a wooden spoon or spatula to gently press against the leaves and twist. This will slightly bruise the leaves and release their flavor—no need to smash them into bits!

Add the blueberries to the container and muddle as you did the mint, just enough to release their juices.

Top off the container with water, stir again, and chill. You can drink this right away, but the flavor intensifies as it soaks, so we recommend letting it sit for a couple of hours or even overnight. Serve as-is over ice or use a fine-mesh strainer to sieve out the fruit and herb bits.

COLD SOUPS

Our cold soups offer a refreshing counterpoint to our hot soups. Enjoy them—at the recommended serving size—as a midmorning pick-me-up in place of a nut milk snack or as a midday reboot.

CUCUMBER-GRAPE-HONEYDEW
CHILLED SOUP (OUR "REFRESH")

This raw soup gets its refreshing appeal from cucumbers, which are known to regulate body temperature, flush out toxins, revive the eyes, and majorly hydrate. Combined with coconut milk, green grapes, lemon, lime, and dill pollen, this soup beautifies the skin, helps regulate blood pressure, supports weight loss, and promotes a healthy heart. When cleansing, we recommend working this in as an afternoon snack or for post-workout recovery. Drink this just like you would a smoothie out of a glass.

YIELD: 6 cups
CLEANSE SERVING SIZE: 12 ounces
PREP TIME: 10 minutes

2 pounds English cucumbers
1 medium honeydew melon (about 2 to 2½ cups), skinned and sliced
½ pound green grapes
2 ounces (about 4 tablespoons) organic coconut milk (preferably Natural Value brand)
1¼ teaspoons fresh lemon juice
2½ teaspoons fresh lime juice
Optional: 1 pinch dill pollen, to taste
Optional: 1 pinch sea salt, to taste

Combine all ingredients in a blender except for the dill pollen and sea salt. Puree on high until smooth, 1 to 2 minutes.

Season to taste with dill pollen and sea salt, if using. Combine on low in blender.

PINEAPPLE, PAPAYA, AND
FENNEL COLD SOUP (OUR "BREATHE")

Tropical pineapple and papaya are packed with vitamins A and C, as well as antioxidants that invigorate and restore your lungs, heart, stomach, colon, and digestive and immune systems. These powerful ingredients scrub your blood cholesterol and provide restorative electrolyte support post-workout or any time of day. We recommend including this chilled soup in your cleanse as an afternoon snack or for post-workout recovery. Drink this just like you would a smoothie, right out of a glass.

YIELD: 6 cups
CLEANSE SERVING SIZE: 12 ounces
PREP TIME: 10 minutes

1 large fennel bulb, quartered
1 medium ripe pineapple (2 to 2½ cups), skinned and sliced
1 unripe papaya (¼ to ½ cup), seeded, skinned, and sliced
1 cup organic and raw coconut water, not from concentrate
1¼ teaspoons fresh lime juice
1¼ teaspoons fresh lemon juice
1 teaspoon lime zest
Pinch sea salt, to taste

Remove the fronds from the fennel bulb. To avoid their slightly bitter taste, we don't use the fronds here, but they contain as much nutrition as the bulb, so we recommend storing them in the freezer, along with any leftover fennel, to use in our Chicken Broth (page 141) or Roasted Vegetable Broth (page 143).

Add all the ingredients to a blender, except the lime zest, 1½ cups water, and salt. Blend on high until smooth, 1 to 2 minutes.

Add the lime zest, water, and salt to taste and combine on low.

CLASSIC GAZPACHO

This gazpacho recipe is light and fresh and super-delicious. If you are looking for a light, cold lunch soup, you have come to the right place. We love the sweet and savory crunch of the vegetables—so no pureeing here. Just chop the veggies, add some sherry vinegar and tomato juice, and you're in heaven. We like to kick it up a notch by adding a dash of Tabasco and a pinch of cayenne or chili powder.

Tomatoes are rich in lycopene, which helps prevent heart disease, cancer, diabetes, age-related eye degeneration, osteoporosis, and aging skin. (It actually acts as an internal sunscreen that protects your skin from sunburn!) Bell peppers are rich in vitamin C (they have twice that of an orange) and the antioxidant mineral manganese, as well as a host of phytonutrients. This soup calls for some advance prep work, but if you make it in the evening, you can have it the next day as a chilled morning or afternoon booster or lunch.

YIELD: 4 to 6 cups
CLEANSE SERVING SIZE: 12 ounces
INACTIVE PREP TIME: 24 hours; **ACTIVE PREP TIME:** 15 minutes

1½ medium beefsteak tomatoes
1 small or ½ medium cucumber, peeled and diced into ¼-inch pieces
1 medium red bell pepper, halved, seeds removed, diced into
    ¼-inch pieces
½ small sweet Vidalia onion, minced
1 medium garlic clove, minced
1 teaspoon Tabasco
⅓ cup sherry vinegar
1 teaspoon sea salt
½ teaspoon fresh black pepper
Optional: Pinch cayenne or chili powder, to taste
2 cups tomato juice
Optional: 1 tablespoon finely chopped fresh cilantro, for garnish
Optional: ½ lime, sliced in wedges, for garnish

Core the tomatoes by running the tip of your knife around the tough spot where the stem meets the flesh. Discard. Chop the tomatoes into ¼-inch pieces.

Add the tomatoes, cucumber, bell pepper, onion, and garlic to a large mixing bowl. Toss with Tabasco, sherry vinegar, salt, pepper, and cayenne, if using.

Let chill overnight or at least 4 hours.

Add the tomato juice. Adjust the seasoning to taste and toss.

Serve in bowls or cups and garnish with cilantro and lime, if desired.

RAW GREEN COMFORT

Thank avocado for this creamy, satisfying "yogurt" soup (which is completely non-dairy). But silky texture isn't its only benefit—avocado is loaded with heart-healthy fats, fiber, and more potassium than bananas. The American Heart Association has published that eating an avocado daily can lower your cholesterol levels and benefit overall health.[1] Add that to the iron, folate, and vitamins B, C, E, and K from spinach, bell peppers, and zucchini, and you have a nutrient-dense treat that's perfect for snacking. We recommend having this creamy treat during your cleanse for an afternoon (or anytime) snack.

YIELD: 3½ cups
CLEANSE SERVING SIZE: 6 ounces
PREP TIME: 15 minutes

1½ cups fresh-squeezed orange juice
¼ cup fresh-squeezed lemon juice
1 ripe or semi-ripe avocado, peeled and pitted
1½ cups baby spinach
1½ cups roughly chopped zucchini
2 medium-spiced chili peppers, or 1 teaspoon red pepper flakes
2 garlic cloves
1 teaspoon fresh grated ginger
1 teaspoon sea salt
Optional: ¼ cup Italian flat-leaf parsley
4 scallions, sliced
¼ teaspoon paprika, for garnish

Add the orange and lemon juices to a blender, followed by the avocado, spinach, zucchini, peppers or pepper flakes, garlic, ginger, salt, parsley (if using), and half the scallions.

Blend until smooth, 1 to 2 minutes.

Adjust seasoning or consistency, if desired—adding a little water, salt, or pepper—and reblend if needed.

Pour into bowls and garnish with the remaining sliced scallions and paprika.

HOT SOUPS

These soups form the foundation of our cleanses. They're what you'll be enjoying for lunch and dinner, and we love that they offer a quick, easy heat-and-eat solution for days when sitting and eating just isn't an option. These recipes run the gamut from the refreshing to the downright sinful. Who knew that comfort food could be so healthy?

Lunch Soups versus Dinner Soups

We've noted which of these soups we recommend to have during your cleanse for lunch, and which for dinner (and which work well for both). Since your cleanse mornings are pretty full of food—with an infused water, broth, and a Superhero—we like having a lighter soup for lunch and reserving the light but more filling options for dinner. You might be thinking, *But isn't eating a heavier meal at night than in the afternoon the opposite of what you normally recommend?* Not at all. Even our heartiest soups are still a very light meal option, meaning they won't tax the digestive system and keep it working overtime when it should be resting at night. Once you transition to post-cleanse eating, feel free to have any of our hot soups at any time of the day.

PUMPKIN MISO SOUP

Miso, kombu, and shiitake mushrooms have been used as traditional remedies for centuries thanks to their ability to fight disease and infection. Teamed up with fiber-full kabocha pumpkin and inflammation-fighting ginger root, they lend supportive nutrients for your circulatory, respiratory, and immune functions. You can easily substitute any hard-skinned winter squash—like butternut, acorn, sweet dumpling, or red kuri—and still reap a huge nutritional gain. This soup is one of our staples— it takes some time to make, but it's worth it! Have it as a heavier lunch or dinner.

Just be sure you're buying live-enzyme miso (the kind sold in the refrigerated case of the grocery store), otherwise you're not going to get its full health benefits.

YIELD: 6 servings
CLEANSE SERVING SIZE: 16 ounces
PREP TIME: 30 minutes; **COOK TIME:** 2½ to 3 hours

3 cups peeled and sliced kabocha pumpkin (from 1 medium pumpkin)
1 (2- to 4-inch) piece of kombu
½ cup shiitake mushroom caps, cut into ½-inch slices
3 teaspoons low-sodium tamari
1 tablespoon minced ginger
1 tablespoon coconut sugar
2 tablespoons miso paste, preferably white or yellow

Preheat the oven to 350°F.

Wrap the pumpkin in foil and bake until tender, about 40 minutes. Be careful not to burn. Set aside.

Make kombu broth by adding 3½ cups water to a small saucepan and heating it over medium-low heat. When it comes to a gentle simmer, add the kombu. Allow the broth to simmer gently for 1 hour. Remove from heat and strain out the kombu into a measuring cup. If any water has evaporated, add more so there are 3½ cups. Set aside.

Add the shiitake mushrooms to a saucepan with the tamari and ¼ cup water and cook over medium-low heat (do not boil) for 1 hour. Add more water if necessary to keep the mushrooms from burning. Set aside.

Combine the pumpkin, kombu water, ginger, coconut sugar, and miso paste in a blender and blend over high speed until smooth, 1 to 2 minutes.

Fold in the cooled mushrooms. Eat immediately or pour into a glass container, cool, and refrigerate.

RED LENTIL AND CARAMELIZED ONION SOUP

High-fiber lentils promote heart health, lower cholesterol, provide vegetable protein, stabilize blood sugar, and are rich in iron and B vitamins. We love combining these earthy gems with the deep, roasty, slightly sweet flavor of caramelized onions. This soup will gently warm your stomach and keep you satisfied.

YIELD: 4 to 6 servings
CLEANSE SERVING SIZE: 16 ounces
PREP TIME: 25 minutes; **COOK TIME:** 30 minutes

2 tablespoons extra-virgin olive oil

3 shallots, diced

4 cloves garlic, chopped

3 carrots, diced

½ teaspoon turmeric powder

½ teaspoon cinnamon

2 yellow beets, peeled and diced

6 cups Roasted Vegetable Broth (page 143) or store-bought low-sodium (MSG-free, gluten-free) version

1¼ cups red lentils

1 teaspoon sea salt, plus more to taste

¼ teaspoon pepper, plus more to taste

1 yellow onion, thinly sliced

10 cardamom pods, or 1½ teaspoons ground cardamom

½ teaspoon coriander powder

Heat a medium-sized saucepan over medium-high heat and add 1 tablespoon of olive oil. When it dances, add the shallots, garlic, carrots, turmeric, and cinnamon. Cook until the shallots soften and the mixture becomes aromatic, 3 to 5 minutes.

Add the beets and vegetable broth and bring the mixture to a boil. Add the lentils and reduce the heat to a simmer. Season with salt and pepper and continue cooking at a simmer for 15 to 25 minutes, or until the lentils are soft and the vegetables are tender.

Prepare the caramelized onions while the soup cooks. If using cardamom pods, crush them (the bottom of a pan works nicely) and remove the seeds. Grind the seeds into a powder with a mortar and pestle.

Heat a medium-sized saucepan over medium-high heat, add 1 tablespoon of olive oil, and heat until the oil dances. Add the onion, cardamom, and coriander. Keep the heat high so the onions begin to brown, stirring continuously. If the onions start sticking to the pan, add a bit of water. Continue cooking for 10 minutes or until the onions are caramelized and golden brown. Reduce the heat if necessary to keep them from burning. Season with a pinch of salt and pepper.

Fill bowls with soup and top with a tablespoon of onions and serve, or simply stir the onions into the soup.

CHICKPEA AND SPINACH SOUP WITH SPICY TURNIPS AND CHICKPEAS

Whether you call them chickpeas or garbanzos, you're still going to get all the healthy protein, fiber, vitamins, and minerals that these legumes have. From cutting cholesterol[2] to contributing to more gorgeous skin and hair, they're a must-have on our grocery and soup list.

YIELD: 4 to 6 servings
CLEANSE SERVING SIZE: 8 ounces
PREP TIME: 20 minutes; **COOK TIME:** 35 minutes

3½ tablespoons extra-virgin olive oil

1 yellow onion, chopped

4 garlic cloves, chopped

1 (1-inch) piece ginger, finely chopped

1½ teaspoons cinnamon

6 cups Roasted Vegetable Broth (page 143) or store-bought low-sodium
(MSG-free, gluten-free) version

Juice and zest of 1 lemon

2 (15-ounce) BPA-free cans or Tetra Paks chickpeas, drained and rinsed

8 ounces cherry tomatoes (about 1½ cups), sliced in half

1 teaspoon ground cumin

1 teaspoon fresh ground ginger

1 teaspoon salt, plus more to taste

¾ teaspoon black pepper, plus more to taste

½ teaspoon ground coriander

½ teaspoon smoked paprika

1 medium turnip, peeled and diced

1 cup packed spinach

Preheat the oven to 425°F.

Heat a medium-sized saucepan over medium-high heat, add 1 tablespoon of olive oil, and when it shimmers, add the onion, garlic, ginger, and 1 teaspoon cinnamon. Cook until the onion is soft, about 5 minutes.

Add the vegetable broth, lemon juice and zest, and 2¼ cups chickpeas. Simmer for 10 minutes. Stir in the tomatoes and continue to cook at a simmer, 5 to 6 minutes.

In a small bowl, combine the cumin, ginger, salt, pepper, coriander, paprika, and ½ teaspoon cinnamon.

Add 1 tablespoon of the spice mixture to a medium-sized mixing bowl and toss to coat with the turnip and 1 tablespoon of olive oil.

Line a baking sheet with parchment paper and spread the turnip pieces on the pan. Bake for 10 minutes.

In the same bowl you used to combine the turnips and the spice mixture, add the remaining ¾ cup of chickpeas, 1½ teaspoons of olive oil, and 1 tablespoon of the spice mix. Toss until everything is evenly coated.

Add the chickpeas to the tray with the turnips and return it to the oven. Bake for another 10 minutes.

Just before serving the soup, stir in the spinach and heat for 2 minutes. Adjust seasoning with salt and pepper, if needed. Top with spicy turnips and chickpeas and serve.

There will be leftover spice mixture, which you can store in an airtight container for up to four weeks.

ROASTED RED PEPPER SOUP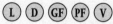

All peppers are good for you, but the very best are the red ones. That's why we created a delicious soup just to highlight these sweet beauties. They are high in vitamins A, C, B_6, and magnesium, making them a great antioxidant source. And with lycopene in the mix, they have been tested in the prevention of many cancers.[3] Now, that's a super-vegetable that has clearly earned its place on our soup list!

This soup makes for a great lunch or light dinner and is delicious served on its own or with our Vegan Parmesan Sprinkles (page 166).

YIELD: 4 to 6 servings
CLEANSE SERVING SIZE: 16 ounces
PREP TIME: 25 minutes; **COOK TIME:** 1 hour

6 red bell peppers, halved, seeds and stems removed
1 tablespoon extra-virgin olive oil, plus more for roasting
2 garlic cloves, roughly chopped
2 shallots, roughly chopped
4 cups Roasted Vegetable Broth (page 143) or store-bought low-sodium (MSG-free, gluten-free) version
1 tablespoon balsamic vinegar
1 tablespoon red wine vinegar
¾ teaspoon salt, plus more to taste
¼ teaspoon red pepper flakes
2 cups Almond Milk (page 148)
Fresh black pepper, to taste
12 to 15 large basil leaves, sliced

Preheat the broiler and line a baking sheet with parchment paper.

Arrange the peppers cut side down on the baking sheet and cover the rounded side with just enough olive oil to coat. Place the peppers under the broiler and cook for 15 to 20 minutes, so the skins are blackened and the peppers are somewhat soft.

Place the peppers in a bowl and cover with plastic wrap, a dish, or a clean towel so they steam for 5 minutes. Remove the cover and let the peppers cool.

When they are cool enough to handle, remove the peppers' skin with your hands. It should slip right off. Transfer the clean peppers directly into the blender.

Heat a medium-sized saucepan over medium heat, add the olive oil, and when it dances, add the garlic and shallots. Cook for about 2 minutes and add the mixture to the blender.

Pour in 1 cup of vegetable broth and puree until smooth, 1 to 2 minutes.

Return the mixture to the saucepan over medium-high heat, add 3 cups vegetable broth, bring to a boil, and then reduce heat to a simmer and cook for 15 minutes.

Add both vinegars, salt, and red pepper flakes. Stir in the almond milk and simmer for 15 minutes more. Remember not to let the mixture boil once the almond milk is added, as it will separate. Taste the soup to see if more vinegar or salt is needed, and add black pepper to taste. Add sliced basil, simmer for 2 minutes, and serve.

ROASTED SQUASH SOUP

Eating fiber-filled squash has been said to help prevent heart disease, high blood pressure, diabetes, and certain types of cancer.[4] It also lends a silky, sumptuous texture to soup that's just the right blend of sweet and savory. Roasting the squash first gives this dish a deeper, richer flavor. You can use any combination of squash for this recipe—kabocha, pumpkin, red kuri, sweet dumpling, and more.

YIELD: 4 to 6 servings
CLEANSE SERVING SIZE: 16 ounces
PREP TIME: 15 minutes; **COOK TIME:** 50 minutes

Extra-virgin olive oil for roasting

2 pounds butternut squash, halved and seeds scooped out

1 pound acorn squash, halved and seeds scooped out

2 teaspoons salt

1 teaspoon pepper

3 garlic cloves

2 medium shallots

½ cup Almond Milk (page 148)

4 cups Roasted Vegetable Broth (page 143) or store-bought low-sodium
    (MSG-free, gluten-free) version

1 tablespoon dried thyme

Preheat the oven to 350°F and line a baking sheet with parchment paper.

Rub just enough olive oil over the flesh of the squash to coat. Sprinkle with
1 teaspoon salt and ½ teaspoon pepper.

Place the squash flesh side down on the baking sheet and bake for 20 minutes or until it is soft. Allow to cool slightly.

Scrape the squash flesh from the skin into a blender. Add the garlic, shallots,
and almond milk. Puree until smooth, 1 to 2 minutes.

Add the puree to a medium-sized saucepan along with the vegetable broth
and bring to a boil. Reduce the heat to a simmer and cook for 15 minutes. Add
the thyme and remaining salt and pepper and continue cooking until the shallot
and garlic have mellowed, about 10 more minutes. Ladle into bowls and serve
immediately.

MINESTRONE

Minestrone soup is simple yet hearty and reminds us of chilly nights around
our family's dinner table. We've taken this traditional dish—which literally
means "big soup"—and really pumped it up with tons of veggies, beans, and
pasta. Plus we added some flavorings that Mom probably wasn't adding to
hers, such as nutty nutritional yeast, which is chock-full of B-complex vitamins,
trace minerals, and all eighteen amino acids. It's excellent for balancing the

systems in the body; converting food to energy; improving memory; minimizing depression, insomnia, nervousness, fatigue, and irritability; and supporting the skin, nails, and hair.

YIELD: 4 to 6 servings
CLEANSE SERVING SIZE: 12 ounces
PREP TIME: 20 minutes; **COOK TIME:** 40 minutes

1 tablespoon extra-virgin olive oil

5 garlic cloves, minced

1 yellow onion, chopped

2 stalks celery, diced

2 teaspoons dried oregano

1 teaspoon dried basil

1 teaspoon fennel seeds, crushed

1 (14-ounce) BPA-free can or Tetra Pak diced tomatoes with juice

4 cups Chicken Broth (page 141), Roasted Vegetable Broth (page 143), or store-bought low-sodium (MSG-free, gluten-free) version

1 chili arbol

1 tablespoon balsamic vinegar

1 tablespoon red wine vinegar

1 teaspoon salt

¾ teaspoon fresh cracked pepper

8 ounces (about 1½ cups) cremini mushrooms, quartered (or cut into smaller bite-sized pieces, depending on size of mushrooms)

1 zucchini, cut into ½-inch pieces

1 yellow squash, cut into ½-inch pieces

1 (15-ounce) BPA-free can or Tetra Pak white beans, drained and rinsed

1 cup packed sliced Tuscan kale

1½ cups rice penne or other gluten-free pasta

1 tablespoon nutritional yeast

¼ cup chopped fresh parsley

Heat a medium-sized saucepan over medium heat, add the olive oil, and heat until it shimmers. Add the garlic, onion, celery, oregano, basil, and fennel seeds and cook until fragrant, about 4 minutes.

Stir in the tomatoes and juice, broth, and chili arbol. Bring the mixture to a boil and then reduce to a simmer. Add both vinegars, salt, and pepper and cook for 20 minutes.

Add the mushrooms, stir, and bring the pot to a boil.

Add the zucchini, squash, beans, kale, pasta, and nutritional yeast and cook at a simmer until the pasta and squash are tender, 5 to 10 minutes. Add the parsley and adjust the seasoning if necessary. Ladle into bowls and serve immediately.

SPRING PEA SOUP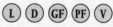

If you like traditional pea soup, you'll love how yummy this vegan, hambone-free version is. This fresh-as-spring soup is rich in phytonutrients, and research shows that green peas help ward off stomach cancer,[5] especially when consumed regularly. Peas have both antioxidant and anti-inflammatory benefits, help regulate blood sugar, and are very high in fiber, omega-3 and omega-6 fats, and vitamin E. You'll need extra time to soak the peas before you prepare this soup, but the advance planning is well worth it.

YIELD: 6 to 8 servings
CLEANSE SERVING SIZE: 8 ounces (lunch) or 12 ounces (dinner)
INACTIVE PREP TIME: 4 hours; **ACTIVE PREP TIME:** 15 minutes;
    COOK TIME: 1 hour

2 cups dried green split peas
1 tablespoon extra-virgin olive oil
2 medium onions, chopped
4 garlic cloves, chopped
6 cups Roasted Vegetable Broth (page 143) or store-bought low-sodium
    (MSG-free, gluten-free) version
½ pound carrots (about 2 large), roughly chopped
2 stalks celery, roughly chopped
¾ teaspoon dried oregano
5 leaves fresh basil
½ teaspoon cumin
¾ teaspoon fresh cracked pepper
2 tablespoons chopped fresh chives, for garnish

Cover the peas in cold water and soak for 4 hours, then drain and rinse.

In a large saucepan or stockpot, heat the olive oil over low heat until it dances and add the onions. Sauté for 5 minutes, then add the garlic and cook for 2 more minutes.

Add the vegetable broth, peas, carrots, celery, oregano, basil, cumin, and pepper. Bring to a boil and then reduce heat to simmer and cover. Cook for 50 minutes, making sure the mixture stays at a simmer.

Pour all ingredients into a blender and puree until thoroughly blended. Add water or more broth to thin out if desired. Garnish with chives and serve.

CREAMY CARROT-GINGER SOUP

Carrots get a bad reputation because of their high sugar content, but did you know that they produce falcarinol, which is shown to reduce your risk of cancer?[6] They are also known to slow down aging and make your skin glow and look healthier with their high levels of beta-carotene. And of course, they are rich in vitamin A, which is good for your vision. That said, we love this soup mostly because of how delicious it is. It's the best, creamiest carrot soup you've ever tasted. If you include it as a meal in your cleanse, choose a broth for your afternoon snack instead of a fruit-based soup.

YIELD: 6 servings
CLEANSE SERVING SIZE: 12 ounces
PREP TIME: 15 minutes; **COOK TIME:** 1 hour and 10 minutes

3 tablespoons extra-virgin olive oil
2 large yellow onions, chopped
1 teaspoon fresh cracked pepper, plus more to taste
10 large organic carrots, cut into ¼-inch pieces
6 cups Chicken Broth (page 141), Roasted Vegetable Broth (page 143), or
    store-bought low-sodium (MSG-free) version
1 inch fresh ginger root, peeled and grated
1 cup fresh-squeezed orange juice
Salt, to taste

Heat a large sauté pan or stockpot over medium heat and add the olive oil. When the oil dances, add the onions, reduce the heat to low, and cover. Cook for about 20 minutes or until the onions are lightly colored and very tender. Stir in the pepper.

Add the carrots and chicken broth to the pot and bring to a boil. Reduce to a simmer and add the ginger. Cover and cook for 25 to 30 minutes so the carrots are very tender.

Transfer the mixture to a blender, add the juice, and blend until completely smooth, 1 to 2 minutes. Add salt to taste.

Return the soup to the pot if you'd like to warm it slightly before eating it right away, or pour it into a glass container and store in the refrigerator for up to three days.

Black Bean Soup

These tasty legumes have long been loved by vegans and vegetarians for all their protein, fiber, antioxidants, and micronutrients. But we think everyone can share in the love. This soup is hearty and savory, and we've added some chipotle peppers to give the beans their own special pizzazz.

YIELD: 4 to 6 servings
CLEANSE SERVING SIZE: 16 ounces
PREP TIME: 10 minutes; **COOK TIME:** 30 minutes

Continued

2 tablespoons extra-virgin olive oil

1 large yellow onion, diced

6 garlic cloves, chopped

1 (14-ounce) BPA-free can or Tetra Pak diced tomatoes with juice

2 chipotle peppers soaked in adobo sauce, sliced in half, sauce reserved
(these can be found in most grocery stores)

4 cups Roasted Vegetable Broth (page 143) or store-bought low-sodium
(MSG-free, gluten-free) version

2 tablespoons red wine vinegar, plus more to taste

1 tablespoon fresh lime juice

1 teaspoon sea salt, plus more to taste

¾ teaspoon fresh cracked pepper, plus more to taste

2 (16-ounce) BPA-free cans or Tetra Paks black beans, drained and rinsed

⅔ cup coarsely chopped fresh parsley

¼ cup coarsely chopped fresh cilantro, for garnish

1 lime, cut into wedges, for garnish

Add the olive oil to a medium-sized pan and heat until it dances. Add the onion and garlic and cook until soft, about 5 minutes.

Transfer the garlic and onion to a blender and add the tomatoes and juice and chipotles. Puree until smooth, 1 to 2 minutes.

Return the tomato mixture to the pan and add the vegetable broth and adobo sauce. Bring to a boil and reduce to a simmer, then cook for 15 minutes. Add the red wine vinegar, lime juice, salt, and pepper. Stir in the black beans and cook 10 minutes more. Add the parsley and adjust the seasoning with salt, pepper, or more vinegar, if desired. Serve garnished with cilantro and lime wedges.

ROASTED EGGPLANT AND LENTIL SOUP

In order to cover all of the vegetable bases, we have created a soup dedicated to eggplant. This beautiful vegetable has been linked to beautifying skin and hair, and has been found useful in the treatment and prevention of

certain cancers.[7] We of course include the gorgeous purple skin in the recipe since research has shown it may contain more fiber than the flesh.

YIELD: 4 to 6 servings
CLEANSE SERVING SIZE: 12 ounces
INACTIVE PREP TIME: 4 hours; **ACTIVE PREP TIME:** 15 minutes;
    COOK TIME: 1 hour and 30 minutes

---

1 cup green lentils, though any other variety would be fine

2 tablespoons extra-virgin olive oil, plus more for pan

1 medium-sized (about ½ pound) Italian eggplant, quartered, skin left on

1 pound fresh Roma tomatoes, quartered

1 large yellow onion, quartered

1 teaspoon sea salt, plus more to taste

½ teaspoon fresh cracked pepper, plus more to taste

1 chili arbol

1 sprig fresh rosemary, plus 2 teaspoons chopped

6 cups Roasted Vegetable Broth (page 143) or store-bought low-sodium (MSG-free, gluten-free) version

2 teaspoons chopped thyme

1 bay leaf

3 carrots, chopped

6 garlic cloves, sliced

Juice and zest of 1 lemon

⅓ cup chopped fresh parsley

Cover the lentils in cold water and refrigerate for 4 hours. Drain, rinse, and set aside.

Preheat the oven to 350°F.

Coat two sheet pans with olive oil.

Place the eggplant on one baking sheet, toss to coat with olive oil (about 1 tablespoon), and arrange them flesh side down. Bake for 20 to 30 minutes.

Arrange the tomatoes and onion on the second baking sheet, toss to coat with olive oil (about 1 tablespoon), and sprinkle with salt and pepper. Roast for 20 to 30 minutes. They should just be beginning to brown.

Add the drained lentils to a medium-sized pot with just enough water to cover by 1 inch. Add the chili, rosemary sprig, and a pinch of salt. Bring to a boil for 10 minutes, reduce to a simmer, and cook until the lentils are soft, 15 to 25 minutes.

When the eggplant, tomatoes, and onion have cooled just enough to handle, roughly chop them all.

If the sheet pans have some caramelized bits stuck to them, pour a little water over the pan and try to loosen them with a whisk or wooden spoon—this has a ton of flavor! Set aside.

Add the chopped vegetables and any pan drippings to a medium-sized saucepan with the vegetable broth, chopped thyme and rosemary, bay leaf, carrots, and garlic. Season with 1 teaspoon salt and ½ teaspoon fresh pepper. Bring to a boil and simmer for 20 minutes.

When the lentils are done, remove the chili and rosemary (not to worry if all that remains is the twiggy stem). Add the vegetable broth mixture, plus the juice and zest of 1 lemon. Cook for another 15 minutes, then check for seasoning and adjust if desired. Just before serving add the chopped parsley.

WHITE BEAN SOUP

White beans, otherwise known as navy beans, are little fiber powerhouses and pack a ton of protein, folate, vitamin B_1, and many minerals, including copper, phosphorus, and iron. They're excellent for stabilizing blood sugar and supporting heart health, while all that B_1 is great for memory.[8] When cooked into a soup, white beans get soft, creamy, and satisfying.

YIELD: 4 to 6 servings
CLEANSE SERVING SIZE: 16 ounces
PREP TIME: 20 minutes; **COOK TIME:** 45 minutes

3 tablespoons coriander seeds

1 tablespoon extra-virgin olive oil

5 garlic cloves, minced

1 medium red onion, chopped fine

2 stalks celery, sliced on an angle into ¼-inch pieces

6 cups Chicken Broth (page 141), Roasted Vegetable Broth (page 143), or
store-bought low-sodium (MSG-free, gluten-free) version

2 (15-ounce) BPA-free cans or Tetra Paks of white beans, drained and rinsed

2 carrots, julienned (a mandoline is ideal here, but by hand is fine too)

8 ounces (about 1 cup) cherry tomatoes, halved

1 teaspoon salt

¾ teaspoon fresh cracked pepper

½ cup parsley, coarsely chopped

¼ cup sliced fresh basil

Zest of 1 lemon

Vegan Parmesan Sprinkles (page 166)

Place the coriander seeds in a small sauté pan over low heat and toast until aromatic, 2 to 3 minutes. Use a spice grinder, mortar and pestle, or back of a pan to grind until fine.

Heat a medium-sized saucepan over medium-high heat and add the olive oil. When it dances, add the coriander, garlic, onion, and celery. Cook for about 3 minutes, or until the onions soften and turn translucent. Add the broth and bring to a boil. Reduce to a simmer and cook for 15 minutes.

Add the white beans to the pot and simmer for 10 minutes. Add the carrots, tomatoes, salt, and pepper. Cook for another 10 minutes. Stir in the parsley, basil, and lemon zest and serve in bowls with a tuft of vegan parmesan sprinkles.

CREAMY TOMATO BASIL SOUP

Of course it is non-dairy, non-GMO, and the most delicious tomato soup you can make (or buy from Soupure). High in fiber, low in calories, and fat free, tomatoes are rich in vitamins A, C, K, and B$_6$, folate, magnesium, potassium, phosphorous, and copper!

YIELD: 6 servings
SERVING SIZE: 12–16 ounces for souping
PREP TIME: 40 min; **COOK TIME:** 35 minutes

2 pounds Roma tomatoes
3 tablespoons extra-virgin olive oil
1½ teaspoon sea salt
1 teaspoon fresh cracked pepper
4 garlic cloves, minced
2 large yellow onions, peeled and chopped
2 carrots, roughly chopped
2 stalk celery, roughly chopped
4 cups Roasted Vegetable Broth (page 43) or store-bought low-sodium
   (MSG-free, gluten-free) version
2 bay leaves
½ cup fresh basil

Preheat oven to 400°F.

Cut tomatoes into chunks, being careful to retain the juice. Place the juice in a bowl for later use. Place the cut-up tomatoes on a baking sheet, and drizzle ¾ of the extra-virgin olive oil over the tomatoes and sprinkle with sea salt and fresh cracked pepper. Place in the center of a preheated oven and cook for 35–45 minutes. Do not let the tomatoes become black, and if they are roasting too quickly, reduce temperature. The longer roasting time helps ensure a sweet taste.

Place the remaining olive oil in a large sauté pan or skillet and heat (you just need enough to coat the bottom of the stock pan). When heated, added the onions and cook for 10 minutes. Then add the chopped garlic and cook for another 4–5 minutes. The garlic should not be brown. If browning, add a tablespoon of water. Then combine in carrots, celery, vegetable broth, bay leaves, basil, and the juice from the tomatoes that you set aside. Simmer for 20 minutes. Add in the roasted tomatoes, and simmer for another 20 minutes.

Remove the bay leaves and combine all ingredients into a Vitamix or blender. Blend till thoroughly pureed. Transfer to a pot to reheat, and serve in bowls. This soup will last about five days in your refrigerator.

EGGPLANT PARMESAN

Another way to use our tomato basil soup is as a delicious stand-in for marinara sauce. We particularly love it smothered over vitamin K–rich eggplants (excellent for circulation, brain health, stabilizing blood sugar, and lowering cholesterol—plus lots of fiber and other nutrients when you leave the skin on), sprinkled with gluten-free breadcrumbs and our vegan parmesan sprinkles, then baked until bubbling and golden.

YIELD: 4 servings
CLEANSE SERVING SIZE: 6 ounces
INACTIVE PREP TIME: 30 minutes; **ACTIVE PREP TIME:** 30 minutes;
   COOK TIME: 40 minutes

2 medium to large eggplants, sliced into ½-inch rounds
2 teaspoons sea salt
3 large eggs
2 cups gluten-free panko breadcrumbs
2 to 3 tablespoons extra-virgin olive oil, plus more for pan
3 cups Creamy Tomato Basil Soup (page 135) or store-bought marinara
   sauce
1 teaspoon fresh oregano
1 cup Vegan Parmesan Sprinkles (page 166) or store-bought vegan
   parmesan cheese
½ teaspoon fresh ground pepper
Spinach
1 tablespoon chopped flat-leaf parsley

Preheat the oven to 400°F.

Place the eggplant rounds on a paper towel–lined baking sheet in a single layer and sprinkle liberally with sea salt, about 1 teaspoon. This will help draw out any bitterness from the eggplant. Lay another paper towel over the top and transfer the eggplant to the refrigerator for 30 minutes.

Prepare your eggplant-dredging stations by whisking the eggs in a wide, shallow bowl or pie dish and placing the breadcrumbs in another. Dip each eggplant round first into the egg wash and then into the breadcrumbs to coat completely. Place them on a baking sheet. Set aside.

Prepare another baking sheet by greasing it with just enough olive oil to coat.

Heat 1 tablespoon of olive oil in an iron skillet or sauté pan over medium heat. When the oil shimmers, gently add the eggplant to the pan and cook until golden brown, about 2 minutes per side (it doesn't need to be cooked through). You may need to add more oil as the eggplant will absorb it.

Arrange the eggplant in a single layer on the greased baking sheet. Slather 2 cups of the tomato basil soup or marinara over the eggplant and sprinkle with oregano, parmesan sprinkles, and ground pepper.

Bake for 30 minutes. In a small pot over medium heat, warm the remaining tomato basil soup or marinara.

Just before serving, heat a teaspoon of extra-virgin olive oil in a cast-iron or sauté pan. Place all the spinach in the sauté pan and gently fold to heat but not wilt the spinach—barely 1 minute of total cook time. Place the spinach in the center of a serving dish and top with eggplant slices, taking care to keep them saucy side up. Spoon the tomato sauce over the eggplant, leaving extra on the side for dipping. Sprinkle with parsley and serve.

Note: 1 pound of gluten-free linguini can be substituted for spinach for flavor preference, but that will increase the calorie count.

CAULIFLOWER LEMONGRASS SOUP

Cauliflower is such a powerful addition to healthy eating that we have created a delicious and light soup around it. This powerhouse has been linked to cancer risk reduction, better digestion, and a healthy heart, and its anti-oxidants and B vitamins are anti-inflammatory.

We love that when cauliflower is cooked until tender, it has a naturally creamy texture that's rich and earthy in flavor.

YIELD: 2 to 4 (8-ounce) servings
CLEANSE SERVING SIZE: 16 ounces
PREP TIME: 10 minutes; **COOK TIME:** 25 minutes

---

1 (1½-inch) piece fresh ginger, peeled and coarsely chopped

4 garlic cloves, coarsely chopped

1 medium shallot, coarsely chopped (about ¼ cup)

1 to 2 Thai chilies, stems removed and halved

2 stalks lemongrass, tough outer leaves removed, bottom trimmed, and cut into 3-inch pieces

1 tablespoon extra-virgin olive oil

6 cups Chicken Broth (page 141), Roasted Vegetable Broth (page 143), or store-bought low-sodium (MSG-free, gluten-free) version

2 fresh kaffir lime leaves, torn

1½-pound head of cauliflower, stem removed and cut into quarter-sized florets

8 ounces (about 1 cup) cherry tomatoes, halved

1 teaspoon fresh-squeezed lime juice

¾ teaspoon coconut sugar, plus more to taste

8 leaves Thai basil, sliced

Salt and pepper, to taste

Place the ginger, garlic, shallot, Thai chilies, and lemongrass in a food processor or blender and pulse until the mixture has a coarse texture. Don't overblend or you could blow out your motor.

Heat a large saucepan over medium-high heat and add the olive oil. When it dances, add the mixture from the blender. Reduce the heat to medium and cook, stirring constantly, until the mixture releases some of its moisture and becomes aromatic. Do not brown.

Pour in the chicken broth and bring to a boil, then reduce to a simmer. Add the kaffir lime leaves and simmer for 15 minutes.

Strain the broth through a mesh strainer, taking care to press all the moisture from the spice paste. Return the strained broth to a saucepan and bring to a boil. Add the cauliflower and tomatoes and simmer until tender, about 5 minutes.

Add the lime juice, the coconut sugar, and the Thai basil. Taste and adjust the seasoning with salt, pepper, and coconut sugar to your liking.

BROTHS

We took Grandma's formula for health and transformed it into an even more powerful remedy. At its most basic, bone broth is made by simmering the bones of almost any vertebrate (typically beef, poultry, lamb, or fish) in water for a long time (we let our bones simmer anywhere from 4 to 6 hours) with vegetables and herbs. But the benefits of bone broths are beyond simple. They're full of glycosaminoglycans (GAGs), which are beneficial to bone, hair, skin, and nail health. Bone broth also contains gelatin, which helps heal the gut lining, reduce inflammation, support healthy skin, and even reduce cellulite. Thanks to these benefits, these broths effectively restore the body during periods of intense healing without adding the stress of digesting solids, such as post-surgery and after uncomfortably symptomatic illnesses. We have found drinking bone broth daily to support your health to be highly beneficial. There's a good reason why people say bone broth is nature's magic elixir! Sip some to start your morning, or toss in your own magical ingredients for a spectacular lunch or dinner.

CHICKEN BROTH

Chicken bone broth is one of the oldest healing traditions in the world and is best known for its protection against colds and flus. Studies have also shown that it may reduce joint pain and inflammation while regenerating hair, skin, bones, and nails.[9] It doesn't get more soothing than this.

YIELD: 6 servings
CLEANSE SERVING SIZE: 12 ounces
PREP TIME: 45 minutes; **COOK TIME:** 4 to 6 hours

1 pound, 6 ounces of chicken bones (we use a combination of gelatin-rich chicken shoulders and feet)
1 to 2 tablespoons balsamic vinegar
1 tablespoon extra-virgin olive oil
½ medium yellow onion, roughly chopped
¼ cup roughly chopped fennel (stalks and fronds are great to use here)
¼ cup roughly chopped carrots
¼ cup roughly chopped celery
1½ teaspoons sea salt
1 bunch parsley
1 (1-inch) piece of kombu

Place the bones in a large pot and cover with 9 cups of water. Add the balsamic vinegar and bring to a boil.

While the water is coming to a boil, heat the olive oil over medium heat in a large sauté pan. Add the onion, fennel, carrots, and celery and cook for 5 minutes. Add the onion mixture to the pot when the water boils, along with the sea salt, parsley, and kombu.

Reduce the heat to a simmer and cook for at least 4 hours or for as long as 6 hours.

Using a colander or sieve, strain all the liquid from the solid pieces. Discard the solid pieces.

Refrigerate the broth overnight. When you remove it from the fridge, remove as much of the fat cap as you like.

Divide into freezer-safe containers for storage and freeze, or refrigerate and consume within five days. Always let broth cool before refrigeration or freezing.

Miso Power-Up

Adding miso to your morning broth is a great way to sneak in all the benefits of this incredible superfood. As we mentioned earlier in the book, miso is fermented soybean paste. Unlike processed soy and its negative health effects, pure soy—and especially fermented soy—has healing abilities when eaten in small amounts. These include restoring beneficial probiotics to the intestines, strengthening the quality of the blood and lymph fluid, reducing the risk of breast, prostate, lung, and colon cancers, protecting against free radicals and radiation, energizing the body, and stimulating the secretion of digestive fluids in the stomach (which is especially important first thing in the morning).[10]

In order to harness miso's full power, make sure to buy a live-enzyme version, which you'll find in the refrigerated aisle in the grocery store. To add miso to your broths, simply whisk in a teaspoon of miso paste for every three cups of liquid, then simmer for 10 minutes. Be sure the soup does not reach a boil, as high heat will kill the miso's live enzymes.

RICHEST BEEF BONE BROTH EVER

You can feel this rich and savory broth right down to your bones. Its minerals support the immune system, while healing compounds like collagen, proline, glycine, and glutamine detoxify, nourish, and soothe. Beef broth has been used as a medicinal remedy for centuries, known among the wise to ease joint pain and arthritic ailments while offering a good dose of collagen for ultimate skin and hair beautification.

YIELD: 1 gallon
CLEANSE SERVING SIZE: 12 ounces
ACTIVE PREP TIME: 20 minutes; **COOK TIME:** 1 to 3 days

3 pounds beef knuckles and shoulder bones

1 pound beef (can be tri-tip or chuck, cut into cubes)

3 large carrots, halved lengthwise

2 medium yellow onions, quartered

1 leek, greens removed, halved lengthwise, and rinsed

3 stalks celery, halved

5 garlic cloves, halved

Optional: Red wine

2 tablespoons black peppercorns

2 tablespoons apple cider vinegar

2 bay leaves

Preheat the oven to 350°F.

Place the bones, beef, carrots, onions, leek, celery, and garlic on a baking sheet and brown for 60 to 75 minutes, or until the vegetables, meat, and bones are deeply browned but not burnt.

Transfer the roasted bones, meat, and vegetables to a large stockpot. Be sure to include all the pan juices, adding a small amount of water or red wine to the hot pan to help loosen any bits that are stuck to the pan. Cover with 6 quarts of cold water. Add the peppercorns, cider vinegar, and bay leaves. Bring the mixture to a boil, reduce to a simmer, and cover. Cook for as few as 24 hours or as long as 3 days over very low heat. The longer you simmer, the deeper the flavor. If the water does not fully cover the vegetables, meat, and bones, add more.

Use a colander or sieve to strain out the solids and discard. Divide into freezer-safe containers for storage and freeze, or refrigerate and consume within five days. Always let broth cool before refrigerating or freezing.

ROASTED VEGETABLE BROTH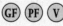

While this isn't technically a bone broth, it is still deeply healing and a very suitable alternative for people who don't eat meat. Mineral-rich vegetable broth is a powerful alkalizing force since it is full of rebalancing minerals and electrolytes. It's also the most delicious and luxurious-tasting vegetable broth we've ever tasted, making it perfect for vegetarians and meat lovers alike.

YIELD: 2¾ quarts (about 11 cups)
CLEANSE SERVING SIZE: 12 ounces
PREP TIME: 20 minutes; **COOK TIME:** 2 hours and 15 minutes

---

4 large carrots, halved lengthwise

2 stalks celery, halved

1 fennel bulb, sliced into thirds

3 large onions, cut into thick slices

8 garlic cloves

2 zucchini, halved

4 shiitake mushrooms, wiped clean and halved

1 large parsnip, halved lengthwise

1 to 2 tablespoons extra-virgin olive oil

1 teaspoon sea salt

½ teaspoon black peppercorns

½ teaspoon red peppercorns or red pepper flakes

2 bay leaves

A few sprigs each of Italian parsley, oregano, and thyme

1 sheet of kombu

Preheat the oven to 350°F.

Combine the carrots, celery, fennel, onions, garlic, zucchini, mushrooms, and parsnip in a large mixing bowl. Drizzle the olive oil over them and toss to coat evenly.

Arrange the vegetables in a single layer on baking sheets and roast for 30 minutes in the center of the oven. Rotate the vegetables on the pan and bake for another 30 to 40 minutes. They should be deeply caramelized and brown, but not burnt.

Transfer the vegetables to a large stockpot. Be sure to add all their juices as well, adding a small amount of water to the hot baking sheet to help loosen any bits that are stuck. Cover with 3 quarts of water and add the sea salt, peppercorns, and bay leaves.

Bring the broth to a boil and reduce to a simmer. Add the herbs and kombu. Simmer uncovered for 1 hour.

Use a colander or sieve to strain out the solids and discard. Divide into freezer-safe containers for storage and freeze, or refrigerate and consume within five days. Always let broth cool before refrigerating or freezing. Can last in the freezer for up to three months.

BROTH BLENDS

Not that our broths aren't delicious enough all by themselves, but we've found that they make the perfect blank canvas for an almost endless number of broth-based soups. Whether it's crunchy, meaty, veggie, spicy, sweet, or savory that you're craving, starting with a simple broth and laying in add-ins is pretty much the easiest (and healthiest) way to create a fulfilling, hearty meal. We've given you some of our favorite combinations and additions, but we highly encourage you to create your own.

CLEANSE SERVING SIZE: 16 ounces (but do not add grains, legumes, or potatoes)

Spring Greens: Sauté garlic and onions in extra-virgin olive oil until translucent, 3 to 4 minutes. Add fresh or frozen peas, asparagus (tough bottoms trimmed and cut into 1-inch pieces on the diagonal), and leeks (white and green parts, thinly sliced) and cook until just beginning to get tender, then simmer in broth until the vegetables have softened. Add a big handful of baby spinach leaves just before serving, and season with sea salt to taste.

Freshly Fennel: Sauté thinly sliced fennel and garlic in extra-virgin olive oil until tender, 2 to 4 minutes. Add thickly sliced carrots and cook until they're just beginning to get tender, then simmer in broth until the vegetables have softened. Season with sea salt to taste.

Clean and Classic: Simmer diced or sliced onion, carrots, and celery in broth until tender. Season with sea salt to taste.

Satisfying Stir-Ins:

- Cooked, shredded chicken
- Cubed and roasted sweet potatoes; squash; root vegetables like beets, parsnips, or celery root
- Grains like cooked quinoa, farro, or gluten-free noodles
- Legumes like cooked lentils, white beans, or black beans
- Fresh herbs like parsley, thyme, basil, mint, cilantro, dill, or rosemary
- Organic tomato paste
- Miso
- Ginger juice
- Fermented beet juice
- Freshly grated turmeric
- Finely chopped chipotle peppers
- Thai red chili paste
- Calabrian chili oil

Tasty Toppers (all of which can also be toppings on our hot soups):

- Diced avocado
- Toasted pine nuts
- Toasted walnuts
- Vegan Parmesan Sprinkles (page 166)
- Sauerkraut
- Crumbled gluten-free crackers (we love Mary's Gone Crackers)
- Crumbled vegetable chips
- Dried fava beans (page 184)

NUT MILKS

Many people who ask us how nut milks are made assume that actual dairy is involved because they're so luxurious and creamy. But that's the beauty of nut milks. They're a delicious and satisfying alternative to dairy milk. And because all you need to make a nut-based milk are the nuts of your choice, water, some natural sweetener, and salt, they are a surefire way to know exactly what you're putting in your body. Unfortunately, we can't say the same for store-bought nut milks. They're typically loaded up with fillers, stabilizers, and preservatives.

We have included two of our favorite nut milk recipes here, but you can make any number of variations using nuts such as cashews, pecans, hazelnuts, walnuts, Brazil, and macadamia by following the same simple method outlined below.

Soaking and Sprouting

You'll notice that our nut milk recipes call for soaking the nuts. This not only makes it easier to process them in the blender and contributes to a smooth, silky consistency, but it's also a way to reap all their nutritional benefits. Truly raw nuts (versus those that have been pasteurized, or heated to kill all the bacteria—good and bad) are loaded with enzymes. However, those enzymes are inhibited by phytic acid, a naturally occurring compound. This makes nuts very difficult to digest and blocks the absorption of minerals, especially iron. In nature, this coating allows seeds and nuts to be eaten by animals and emerge whole, ready to sprout in the soil (instead of breaking down in the animals' guts). Soaking, however, breaks down the phytic acid. Sprouting takes this process one step further and "activates" nuts, or essentially begins the digestion process. By doing this, we are saving our bodies' energy by not taxing them with extra digestion. You can apply these same principles to seeds, legumes, and grains, which all benefit from soaking and/or sprouting.

Our nut milk recipes call for just soaking, since this is a bit easier and less time-consuming than sprouting, while still providing nutritional benefits. If you want to take it a step further, though, here's a simple guide to sprouting:

Fill a quart-sized mason jar one-third full with nuts, seeds, legumes, or grains and cover with water. Place a cheesecloth or nut bag over the mouth of the jar and screw on just the outer ring portion of the lid. Ingredients have different sprouting times, ranging from a few hours to a few days, but there are many online resources with specific times. A few times a day, drain the jar contents through the cheesecloth, rinse, and cover with water once again. Repeat until the desired sprouting is achieved. Store for up to five days in the refrigerator.

ALMOND MILK

Almonds reduce heart attack risk, lower "bad" cholesterol, protect your arteries from damage, build strong bones and teeth, are loaded with healthy fats, aid weight loss, stabilize blood sugar, support brain function, nourish the nervous system, and alkalize the body. Plus, almond milk is creamy and delicious! You'll never want to drink its cow counterpart again!

YIELD: 3 to 4 cups
CLEANSE SERVING SIZE: 12 ounces
INACTIVE PREP TIME: 12 hours; **ACTIVE PREP TIME:** 10 minutes

1 cup raw shelled almonds
1 whole vanilla bean, roughly chopped (or ½ teaspoon vanilla extract)
Optional: 2 dates, pitted
Pinch sea salt
Optional: Pinch cinnamon

Soak the nuts. Place the almonds in a bowl and cover with about 1 inch of water. Let stand, uncovered, overnight or for at least 12 hours. (The longer you soak, the creamier the milk will be!) If necessary, though, it is fine to soak for only 1 to 2 hours.

Drain and rinse the nuts. Drain the almonds in a colander or sieve and rinse them under cool running water (they should feel a little squishy).

Blend. Place the almonds in a high-powered blender with 3½ cups of water and the vanilla bean (or extract) plus the dates, if using them. For almond milk serving as a base to the Superhero (page 151), do not add dates. Blend for about 1 minute on the highest speed. The almonds should be broken down into a fine meal and the water should look white and opaque.

Strain the milk. Place your nut milk bag over a large bowl and separate the almond milk from the almond meal by pouring the almond mixture into the bag. Gently squeeze the bag to get all the milk out (this may take a couple of minutes). If the milk has been drained and you need to add more milk to the bag, be sure to remove the pulp left over before adding more milk to be strained. Reserve the pulp (see note below).

Additional sweeteners/flavor enhancers. Rinse the blender and pour in the strained almond milk. For cleansers drinking the almond milk alone (i.e., not as a base to our Superhero), try adding a handful of organic strawberries to the blender and blend on low until smooth. Add the sea salt and cinnamon, if using, and blend on low for about 1 minute. For almond milk serving as a base to our Superhero, do not add cinnamon. If you want to thin out the milk, add a little water until you reach the desired consistency.

Refrigerate and enjoy. Pour the milk into a glass container and store in the refrigerator for up to three days. Make sure to shake the container before consuming, as the mixture will separate over time.

No Waste Here!

The leftover almond meal can be used many ways—and should be, considering it's just as nutritious as the nuts themselves and high in fiber. Try it in our delicious Nut Pulp Macaroons (page 192) or incorporate it into cookies, homemade granola, or smoothies. It can also be spread on a baking sheet and baked in a low oven until dry (about 2½ hours) to give it a toastier flavor. If you don't want to use the pulp right away, just freeze it and use it later.

Pistachio Milk

Pistachios are excellent for heart health, strengthen your immune system, and have a hearty natural sweetness that's perfect for curbing cravings. They make it easy to go green!

YIELD: 3 to 4 cups
CLEANSE SERVING SIZE: 12 ounces
INACTIVE PREP TIME: 8 to 12 hours; **ACTIVE PREP TIME:** 10 minutes

1 cup raw shelled organic pistachios
1 whole vanilla bean, roughly chopped (or ½ teaspoon vanilla extract)
Pinch sea salt
Optional: 1 teaspoon ground cardamom

Soak the nuts. Place the pistachios in a bowl and cover with about 1 inch of water. Let stand, uncovered, for 8 to 12 hours. (The longer you soak, the creamier the milk will be!) If necessary, though, it is fine to soak for only 1 to 2 hours.

Drain and rinse the nuts. Drain the pistachios in a colander or sieve and rinse them under cool running water (they should feel a little squishy).

Blend. Place the pistachios in a high-powered blender with 3½ cups of water and the vanilla bean (or extract). Blend for about 1 minute on the highest speed. The pistachios should be broken down into a fine meal and the water should look white and opaque.

Strain the milk. Place your nut milk bag over a large bowl and separate the milk from the meal by pouring the pistachio mixture into the bag. Gently squeeze the bag to get all the milk out (this may take a couple of minutes). If the milk has been drained and you need to add more milk to the bag, be sure to remove the pulp left over before adding more milk to be strained. Reserve the pulp (see note on page 149).

Additional sweeteners/flavor enhancers. Rinse the blender and pour in the strained pistachio milk. For cleansers drinking the pistachio milk as-is, try adding a handful of organic blueberries or raspberries to the blender and blend on low until smooth. Add the sea salt and cardamom, if using, and blend on low for about 1 minute. If you want to thin out the milk, add a little water until you reach the desired consistency.

Refrigerate and enjoy. Pour the milk into a glass container and store in the refrigerator for up to three days. Make sure to shake the container before consuming, as the mixture will separate over time.

SUPERHERO

As a creamy smooth, non-dairy nut milk "soup" smoothie, this is our most evolved piece of nutritional artistry yet. Boasting twelve ingredients designed to feed your brain all day, this satisfying solution to hunger does so much more for you than provide superior taste. Made with dried fruits, a collection of nuts and seeds, and a bold combination of super-ingredients like reishi, maca, and cordyceps, this smoothie is perfect for starting your day after a soothing bone broth, reviving a post-workout body, or simply (and healthily) replacing a meal.

YIELD: 6 cups
CLEANSE SERVING SIZE: 12 ounces
INACTIVE PREP TIME: 40 minutes; **PREP TIME:** 20 minutes

1 dandelion tea bag
2 cups Almond Milk (page 148)
½ cup organic coconut milk (Natural Value brand is great as it uses
   no emulsifiers)
7 teaspoons agave
½ cup walnuts
3 whole dried apricots
3 whole pitted dates
5 whole Brazil nuts
7 teaspoons chia seeds
1 teaspoon gelatinized maca root
1 teaspoon reishi powder
1 teaspoon cordyceps powder
Sea salt, to taste

Steep the tea in 3 cups of hot water for 40 minutes and set aside.

Pour the tea, almond milk, coconut milk, and agave into a blender and blend on low just to combine, about 1 minute.

Add the remaining ingredients (except sea salt). Puree on high for 1 to 2 minutes, or until well combined and creamy. You may have to stop the machine periodically to scrape down the sides. You may also need to add a bit more almond milk to get the desired consistency.

Add sea salt to taste and combine on low.

Store in an airtight glass container in the refrigerator for up to 36 hours.

NUT MILK SMOOTHIE ALTERNATIVE FOR CLEANSERS

For cleansers who have nut allergies or just don't want a nut milk as your morning milk or smoothie, replace with a cold soup from pages 115–120. Or for another milky protein-based alternative, replace with a simple smooth and creamy, non-dairy, vegan, nut-free yogurt smoothie made by blending together an organic dairy-free, vegan yogurt (try So Delicious dairy-free cultured coconut milk yogurt from Whole Foods) with a half cup of your favorite berries and your favorite non-dairy, nut-free milk or water (added for desired consistency).

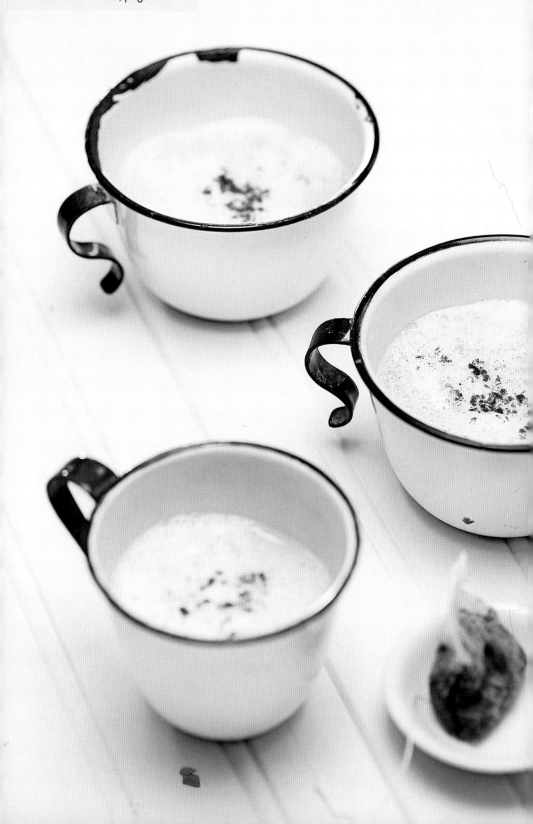

Almond Chai Tea Latte, page 154

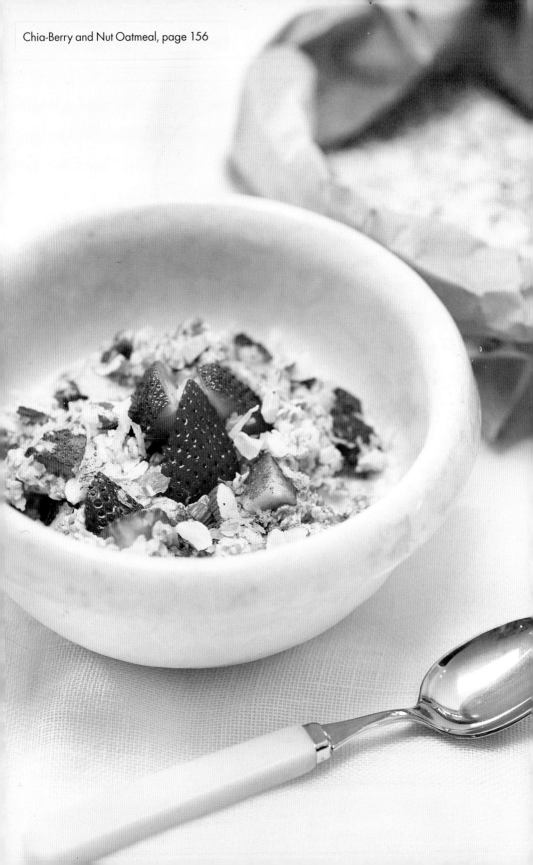

Chia-Berry and Nut Oatmeal, page 156

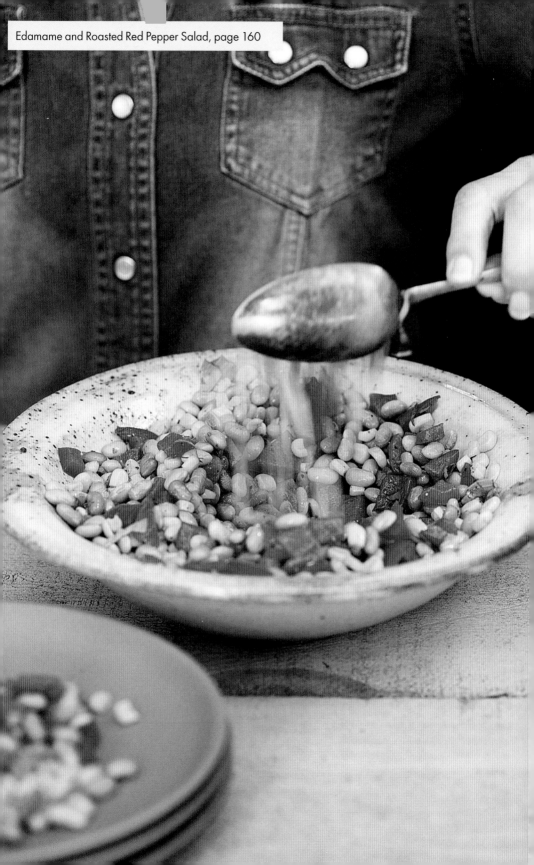

Edamame and Roasted Red Pepper Salad, page 160

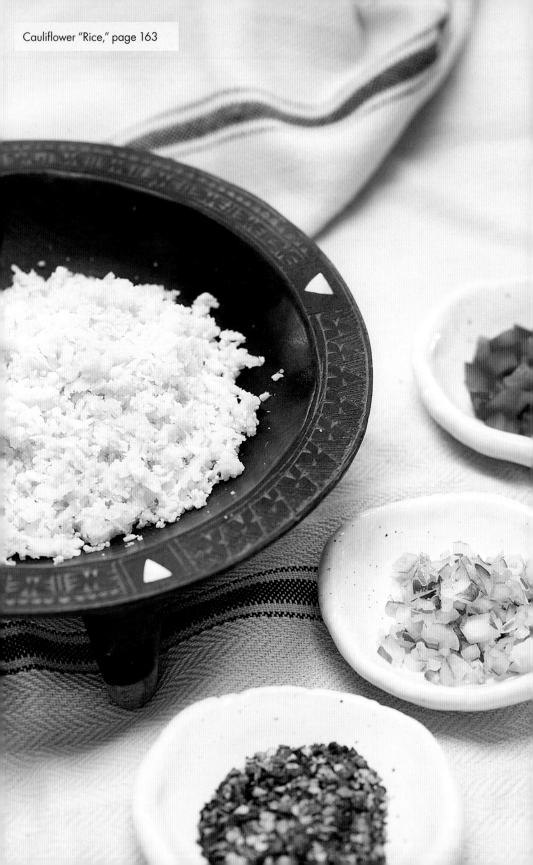

Cauliflower "Rice," page 163

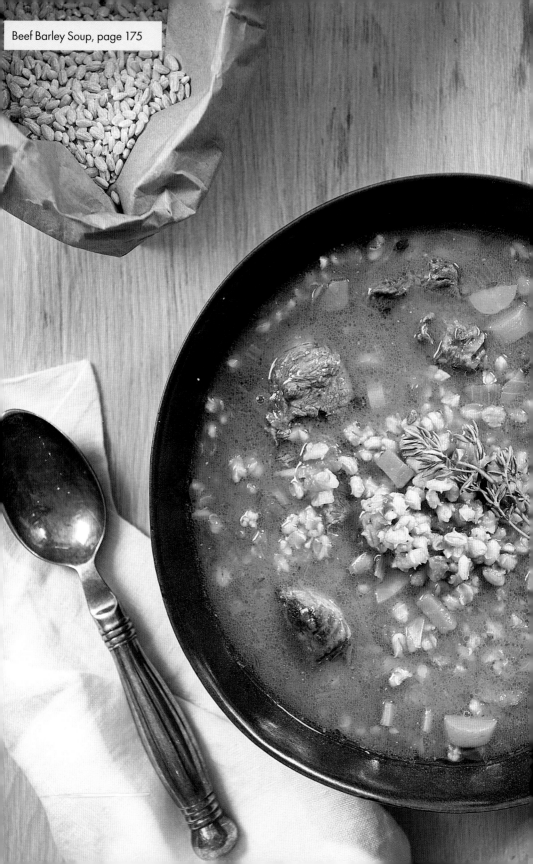

Beef Barley Soup, page 175

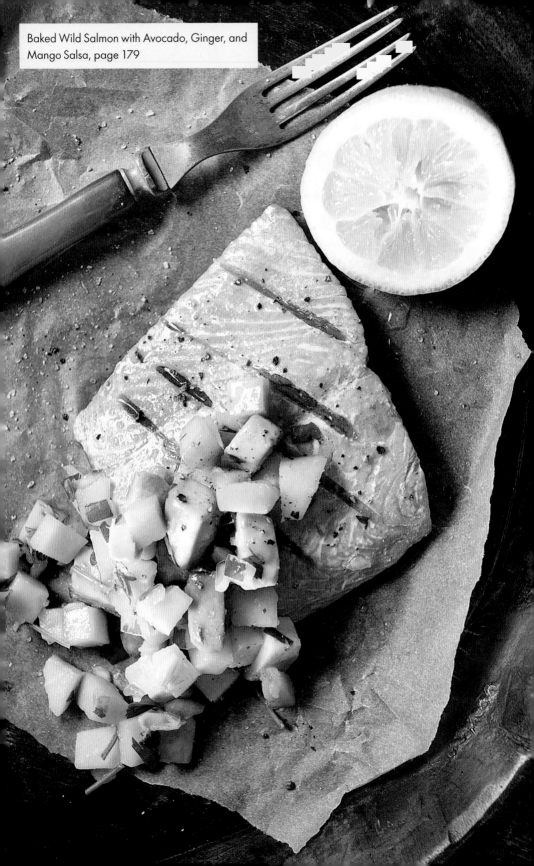

Baked Wild Salmon with Avocado, Ginger, and Mango Salsa, page 179

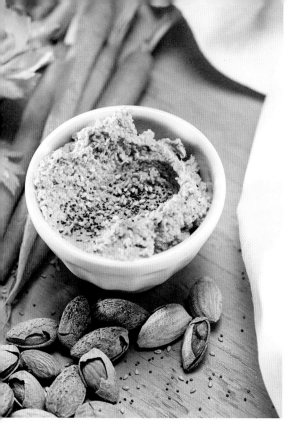

So-Delicious-I-Can't-Believe-It's-Green Dip, a.k.a. Edamame "Hummus," page 186

Blueberry Mojito, page 188

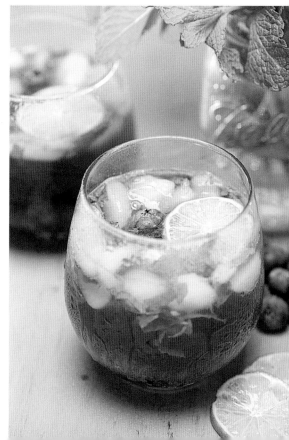

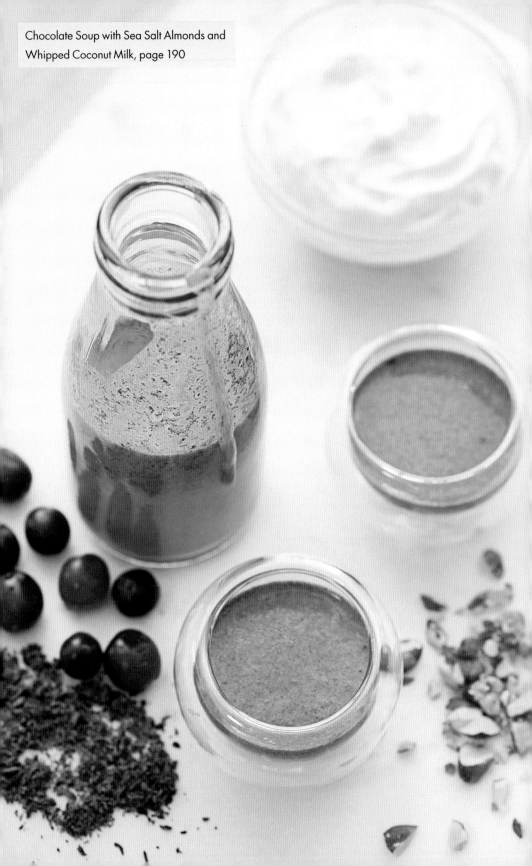

Chocolate Soup with Sea Salt Almonds and
Whipped Coconut Milk, page 190

TEAS AND LATTES

These are treats to enjoy throughout the day, whether you're craving a post-workout treat, a midafternoon break, or a pre-sleep nightcap.

SWEET DREAMS

Turmeric, cardamom, and ginger are Indian spices known for their healing powers, which include being anti-inflammatory, antidepressant, detoxifying, and diuretic, plus being antioxidant-rich. They are also good for warding off bad breath and help calm and relax the body. This sweet milk tea is the perfect soothing treat before bed or on a cold afternoon.

YIELD: 2 servings
CLEANSE SERVING SIZE: 4 to 6 ounces
INACTIVE PREP TIME: 20 minutes to 4 hours;
   ACTIVE PREP TIME: 10 minutes; **COOK TIME:** 2 minutes

2 tablespoons pistachios, almonds, or cashews
2 cups Almond Milk (page 148)
¼ teaspoon ground cinnamon
½ teaspoon fresh grated ginger
¼ teaspoon nutmeg
¼ teaspoon turmeric
¼ teaspoon cardamom
1 teaspoon vanilla extract
1 teaspoon raw honey or agave syrup

Place the nuts in a bowl, cover with about 1 inch of cold water, and let stand for 4 hours. Or, alternatively, soak the nuts in boiling water for 20 minutes. Drain and rinse the nuts.

Add the nuts to a blender with the almond milk. Blend on high until smooth, 1 to 2 minutes. Add the remaining ingredients and blend until fully combined. To enjoy, heat in a saucepan over low heat until just-warmed and not boiling.

ALMOND CHAI TEA LATTE

This tea promotes digestion and fights disease with its high antioxidant levels. It's a delicious and good-for-you alternative to regular chai lattes, which are full of dairy and sugar. To make this a vegan treat, swap out the honey for another natural sweetener such as maple or coconut syrup. Enjoy this drink hot or cold, whenever you need a little "me" time.

YIELD: 2 to 3 cups
CLEANSE SERVING SIZE: 4 to 6 ounces
PREP TIME: 10 minutes; **COOK TIME:** 5 minutes

3½ cups Almond Milk (page 148)
½ teaspoon cinnamon
¼ teaspoon cardamom
½ teaspoon ginger
Optional: Pinch black pepper
3 tablespoons raw honey, maple syrup, or agave
1 Darjeeling tea bag

Combine the milk, cinnamon, cardamom, ginger, and pepper (if using) in a blender and blend on low speed to combine, about 1 minute.

Pour the mixture into a small saucepan and heat over low heat. Add the sweetener and mix to dissolve. Cook until the mixture is just beginning to gently bubble around the edge of the pan.

Add the tea bag and allow it to steep for about 1 minute. Pour into two mugs and enjoy!

Lemon-Ginger Tea

Whether you are warding off the flu or just want a little pick-me-up, this tea is perfect for battling sickness and fatigue. Lemon is packed with vitamins C and B, as well as calcium, iron, magnesium, and potassium, while ginger is known as both an anti-inflammatory and a digestion aid. The two together help cleanse the body, flushing out toxins while filling you up with vitamins and minerals.

YIELD: 2 servings
CLEANSE SERVING SIZE: 6 to 8 ounces
PREP TIME: 15 minutes; **COOK TIME:** 10 minutes

½ lemon, ¼ teaspoon zest reserved
1 (1-inch) piece fresh ginger root, peeled and minced
Raw honey or agave, to taste

In a small saucepan, bring 2 cups of water to a boil. Reduce to a simmer and squeeze in the juice of the lemon half, tossing in the rind too. Add the ginger and simmer for 7 minutes. Stir in honey or agave to taste. Strain and serve in mugs topped with lemon zest.

11

Healthy Pre-, Post-, and Mini-Cleanse Recipes

Whether you're transitioning into or out of a cleanse, substituting a soup for lunch or dinner for a mini-cleanse, or looking for healthier everyday meal options, these recipes are perfect for supplementing our cleanse soups. We've included some of our favorite meal ideas, including some delightfully sinful (but not!) treats.

BREAKFAST

CHIA-BERRY AND NUT OATMEAL

This bowl of goodness is loaded with antioxidants, fiber, and powerful phyto-nutrients that support energy, stamina, and beauty. The vitamin C–rich berries and omega-3-packed chia seeds are a surefire way to enrich your day.

This dish takes no time to whip up in the morning, but an even simpler no-cook option is to combine all the ingredients in a mason jar and store overnight in the refrigerator. Breakfast on the go!

YIELD: 2 servings
PREP TIME: 5 minutes; **COOK TIME:** 10 minutes

⅔ cup gluten-free rolled oats, uncooked
1 cup berries (fresh or frozen)
1 tablespoon chia seeds
1 tablespoon unsweetened coconut flakes
1 tablespoon sliced raw almonds
Optional: Coconut or Almond Milk (page 148), for serving
Optional: ¼ teaspoon raw honey or agave syrup

Combine the oats, berries, chia seeds, and coconut flakes in a small pot with 1½ cups of water and bring to a boil. Reduce the heat and stir occasionally for 5 minutes or until the oats are fully cooked.

Top with sliced almonds, almond or coconut milk, and honey (if desired) and serve.

CINNAMON BERRY SUPERFOOD MUESLI

YIELD: 1 serving
PREP TIME: 5 minutes

½ cup gluten-free rolled oats, uncooked
1 to 2 tablespoons raw nuts such as walnuts, almonds, or pecans, broken into small pieces
1 tablespoon freshly ground flaxseeds or chia seeds
½ cup organic strawberries, raspberries, or blueberries
Optional: 1 tablespoon unsweetened coconut flakes
½ cup coconut or Almond Milk (page 148)
Cinnamon, for serving

Combine the oats, nuts, flaxseeds, berries, and coconut (if using) in a medium mixing bowl. Top with the coconut or almond milk and a sprinkle of cinnamon. Stir to combine and enjoy.

OMELET WITH FARMERS' MARKET VEGETABLES AND ROASTED JAPANESE SWEET POTATO FRIES

Omelets—with the immune-strengthening and brain-boosting effects of choline- and sulfur-rich eggs—are the perfect blank canvas for adding all kinds of seasonal veggies. We kick ours up a notch by adding turmeric, a powerful spice that's associated with anti-inflammatory and antioxidant properties, lowering the risk of heart disease and cancer (and may even help treat cancer), preventing and treating Alzheimer's, mitigating the effects of arthritis and depression, and delaying aging and the onset of chronic disease.[1]

YIELD: 2 servings
PREP TIME: 10 minutes; **COOK TIME:** 10 minutes

4 large eggs
⅛ teaspoon turmeric
Sea salt and pepper, to taste
½ teaspoon extra-virgin olive oil
Handful chopped baby spinach
½ cup halved cherry tomatoes
1 cup asparagus tips, blanched
1 teaspoon fresh herbs such as basil, marjoram, thyme, or chives, chopped
1 batch Roasted Japanese Sweet Potato Fries (recipe follows)

Combine the eggs, turmeric, and a pinch of salt and pepper in a small bowl. Whisk until just blended.

Heat a small frying pan over medium-low heat and add the olive oil, swirling to coat the pan. Add the egg mixture and let cook for about 60 seconds. Add the vegetables and some of the herbs, cook for another 1 to 2 minutes or to desired liking, then fold the omelet in half so the vegetables are wrapped in the egg. Slide onto a plate, cut into two portions, sprinkle with the remaining herbs, and serve with a side of roasted Japanese sweet potato fries.

Roasted Japanese Sweet Potato Fries

Slightly sweeter than American yams, Japanese sweet potatoes are bursting with fiber and vitamin C. They're particularly delicious roasted up into sweet and salty "fries."

YIELD: 2 servings
PREP TIME: 10 minutes; **COOK TIME:** 25 minutes

1 large Japanese sweet potato, peeled, if desired, and cut into long,
   ½-inch-thick strips
1 to 2 tablespoons coconut or extra-virgin olive oil
Dash of sea salt
Optional: 1 teaspoon chopped rosemary

Preheat the oven to 400°F and line a baking sheet with parchment paper.

Toss the sweet potato strips in just enough oil to coat. Arrange them on the baking sheet and sprinkle with salt and rosemary, if desired. Bake for 25 minutes or until golden brown.

SALADS AND VEGGIES

These simple but satisfying dishes can be made meal-sized for the three-day mini-cleanse and are a great way to prepare for a cleanse or to round out your post-cleanse diet. Use them to supplement soups for a gentle reintroduction to solid foods and a healthy ever after.

ROASTED BRUSSELS SPROUTS

Far from the sad, soggy sprouts you ate growing up, these are crunchy and caramelized. Brussels sprouts are high in fiber, riboflavin, magnesium, phosphorus, and copper, as well as vitamins A, B, C, and K. They are amazing for digestive and cardiovascular health, reduce inflammation, provide stellar antioxidant support, and have been proven to provide superior detoxification support thanks to their beneficial compounds.

YIELD: 4 to 6 servings
PREP TIME: 5 minutes; **COOK TIME:** 35 to 40 minutes

1 pound Brussels sprouts
1 teaspoon extra-virgin olive oil
1 teaspoon sea salt
½ teaspoon fresh cracked pepper

Adjust your oven's racks so one is situated in the middle. Preheat the oven to 400°F.

Trim the tough stems from the Brussels sprouts and remove any dead or old leaves. Slice them in half.

In a medium mixing bowl, toss the sprouts with oil, salt, and pepper.

Arrange the Brussels sprouts on a baking sheet so they sit in a single layer. Cook for 20 minutes, then flip. Continue cooking for another 15 to 20 minutes, or until the sprouts are tender and lightly browned.

EDAMAME AND ROASTED RED PEPPER SALAD

We've packed a ton of nutrition into this dish, which makes for a delicious chilled side or salad. Edamame is considered a complete protein, meaning it contains ample amounts of amino acids, the building blocks of protein. It's also loaded with minerals, calcium, iron, phosphorus, and sodium, as well as vitamins A and C. Red peppers are also a nutritional powerhouse. They contain almost 300 percent of your daily vitamin C intake, which, besides being a powerful antioxidant, is necessary for the proper absorption of iron. They're a great source of vitamin B_6 and magnesium, a combination that has been shown to decrease anxiety. B_6 is also a natural diuretic, which can reduce bloating and prevent hypertension. Red bell peppers are high in vitamin A, which is great news for your eyesight, especially night vision. They're also packed with antioxidants that can help prevent many cancers. And last, bell peppers help you burn calories. Recent research has shown that these peppers can boost your metabolic rate without increasing your heart rate and blood pressure.[2] Seconds, anyone?!

YIELD: 6 servings
INACTIVE PREP TIME: 30 minutes; **ACTIVE PREP TIME:** 15 minutes;
   COOK TIME: 20 minutes

---

12 ounces fresh or frozen shelled edamame

1 red bell pepper, halved and seeds removed

1 cup fresh or frozen corn kernels, or substitute 1 cup avocado cut into cubes (cut avocado after you have cooked and cooled other vegetables)

¼ cup finely diced scallion

2 garlic cloves, minced

3 teaspoons extra-virgin olive oil

¾ teaspoon sea salt, plus more to taste

¼ teaspoon fresh cracked pepper, plus more to taste

2 teaspoons balsamic vinegar

¼ teaspoon minced fresh ginger

¼ teaspoon red pepper flakes, plus more to taste

¼ cup finely chopped fresh basil leaves

Preheat the oven to 400°F. Line a baking sheet with foil.

In a large bowl, combine the edamame, red bell pepper, corn, scallion, and garlic, and toss with 2 teaspoons of olive oil, salt, and pepper. If substituting avocado for the corn, do not add the avocado (see page 162).

Spread the mixture on a baking sheet so it sits in a single layer. Bake until the edamame and pepper are starting to brown. Allow to cool slightly.

When you can comfortably handle the pepper, cut into bite-sized pieces.

Place the mixture in a clean mixing bowl and transfer to the refrigerator to chill for 30 minutes.

If substituting avocado for corn, peel and cube the avocado and toss it into the mixture of chilled vegetables with the balsamic vinegar, ginger, red pepper flakes, basil, and 1 teaspoon of olive oil. Adjust the seasoning as desired.

SPINACH SALAD WITH POMEGRANATES, TOASTED WALNUTS, AND LEMON-MUSTARD VINAIGRETTE

You might fall in love with this salad because of how easy and delicious it is—the sweet and juicy pomegranates mixed with earthy spinach, meaty toasted walnuts, and bright lemon-mustard vinaigrette. Or you could be smitten because it's loaded with antioxidant superfoods. A pomegranate provides about 40 percent of the daily vitamin C requirement; spinach is an excellent source of vitamins K and A along with magnesium, folate, manganese, and iron; and walnuts are rich in omega-3 fats, copper, manganese, and biotin. It's the ultimate in health and beauty in a bowl.

YIELD: 4 servings
PREP TIME: 15 minutes; **COOK TIME:** 10 minutes

¼ cup walnut halves
1 (10-ounce) bag fresh spinach
1 pomegranate (about ½ cup seeds)
½ cup Lemon-Mustard Vinaigrette (recipe follows—use only half recipe if cleansing)
Optional: ¼ cup crumbled blue cheese or goat cheese, or 1 tablespoon sunflower seeds

Preheat the oven to 375°F.

Spread the walnuts on a baking sheet and bake for about 10 minutes or until fragrant and lightly browned. Set aside to cool.

Add the spinach, pomegranate seeds, and walnuts to a mixing bowl and toss with lemon-mustard vinaigrette. Serve with a sprinkling of blue cheese, goat cheese, or sunflower seeds, if desired.

Lemon-Mustard Vinaigrette

YIELD: About 1 cup
PREP TIME: 10 minutes

½ cup extra-virgin olive oil
¼ cup red wine vinegar
2 tablespoons Dijon mustard
2 tablespoons fresh-squeezed lemon juice
1 teaspoon raw honey or maple syrup
1 small garlic clove, minced
1 teaspoon dried oregano
½ teaspoon fresh cracked black pepper
½ teaspoon sea salt

Add all the ingredients to a jar with a lid, shake, and serve. Refrigerate leftovers, which will store well for a week.

CAULIFLOWER "RICE"

It can be hard taking unhealthy foods out of your diet, which is why it's important to add in lots of other options that scratch the itch. We love this substitute for white rice, especially because it's a fantastic canvas for a number of different flavor and ingredient variations. Plus it's amazing for your digestion, heart, joints, and overall health. While cauliflower might not taste exactly like white rice, the texture is amazingly similar, making it chewy and satisfying.

So instead of mourning the absence of stripped, depleted, unhealthy white rice, celebrate the new, delicious, fresh, and healthy foods you're giving your body.

Basic Cauliflower Rice: Oven Method

YIELD: 4 to 6 servings
PREP TIME: 10 minutes; **COOK TIME:** 10 to 15 minutes

1 head cauliflower, stem and tough outer leaves removed (yes, that's it!)

Preheat the oven to 425°F.

If necessary, remove any brown or black spots with a paring knife. Cut the cauliflower in half and remove the florets until you are left with the core. Discard the core.

Working in batches, place the florets in a food processor and pulse (or grate with a good old-fashioned grater) until they have the texture of rice—evenly chopped but not pulverized.

Spread the "rice" out on one or more baking sheets so it sits in a single layer. Bake for 10 to 15 minutes, tossing at least once. It's done when the rice is tender and just beginning to brown.

Basic Cauliflower Rice: Frying Pan Method

YIELD: 4 to 6 servings
PREP TIME: 10 minutes; **COOK TIME:** 10 minutes

1 head cauliflower, stem and tough outer leaves removed
1 tablespoon extra-virgin olive oil or safflower oil

If necessary, remove any brown or black spots with a paring knife. Cut the cauliflower in half and remove the florets until you are left with the core. Discard the core.

Working in batches, place the florets in a blender or food processor and pulse until they have the texture of rice—evenly chopped but not pulverized.

In a large non-stick frying pan, heat the olive oil until it shimmers, then add the "rice." Cook for 5 to 7 minutes, stirring frequently and making sure the rice is crispy on the outside but remains tender on the inside.

"Rice" Variations

Classic Onion Rice (frying pan method): Add 1 small diced onion to a frying pan with the oil before adding the rice. Sauté over medium heat until soft and translucent, 4 to 6 minutes. Add rice plus a pinch of sea salt, turn heat up to medium-high, and cook as described above. Other vegetables would be delicious here too: sliced summer squash, chopped broccoli, or spinach.

Chinese Vegetable Fried Rice (frying pan method): Follow the Classic Onion Rice recipe above, adding 1 cup of assorted vegetables after the onions have cooked. Peas (frozen is great), diced carrots, water chestnuts, and bok choy are favorites. Cook until tender, 4 to 6 minutes. Stir in the rice plus 2 to 3 tablespoons of soy sauce (to taste), then cook 5 to 7 minutes more, until the cauliflower is crispy on the outside but tender on the inside.

Lemon Rice (frying pan or oven method): Add juice and zest of 1 lemon to the rice while sautéing or before baking. Cilantro and lemon taste great together, so try adding ¼ cup of chopped cilantro to the finished dish for a little pizzazz (not to mention antioxidants and lead detoxification).

Herbed Rice (frying pan or oven method): Add 1 to 2 tablespoons of hearty fresh herbs such as rosemary, thyme, marjoram, or oregano before sautéing or baking, or more tender herbs such as fresh parsley, basil, cilantro, or chives in the last minute or two of cooking.

Spanish Rice (frying pan method): Add ½ of a diced onion plus 1 diced green pepper, red pepper, and zucchini, and 2 chopped garlic cloves to the frying pan with oil before the rice and sauté over medium heat until heated through, about 5 minutes. Add the rice with ½ cup of your favorite broth. When the cauliflower starts to soften, add 1 (6-ounce) can of organic tomato paste and seasonings to taste (try dried oregano, saffron, paprika, red pepper flakes, and/or salt), and cook over low heat for another 3 to 4 minutes.

"Cheesy" Rice (frying pan or oven method): After you have prepared the rice, mix in our delicious creamy, non-dairy Velvety Cheese Sauce (page 167), to taste, and enjoy!

SAUCES AND TOPPINGS

We all love cheese, whether it's smooth and creamy or salty and tangy. Just about any food gets that much more exciting smothered in the stuff, so we created these non-dairy condiments that you can use on just about anything—meats, vegetables, potatoes, gluten-free pastas, and even our soups. The secret is using nutritional yeast, a complete protein that's an excellent source of fiber and several B vitamins. Now, kids, everyone say, "Cheese!"

Vegan Parmesan Sprinkles

Try this on our White Bean Soup (page 134) or over some green vegetables for a layered, savory flavor.

YIELD: About 1 cup
PREP TIME: 10 minutes; **COOK TIME:** 10 minutes

½ cup pine nuts
½ cup raw almond slivers
1 teaspoon garlic powder
¼ cup nutritional yeast

Preheat the oven to 300°F.

Place all ingredients in the bowl of a food processor. Pulse until the mixture is coarse and resembles grated parmesan cheese. (It is very important not to overblend, because you will create a goopy mess.)

Spread the mixture over a small baking sheet with edges and bake for 10 minutes or until the flakes are evenly brown and aromatic, stirring two or three times to brown evenly.

Allow to cool, and store in an airtight container at room temperature for up to a week.

VELVETY CHEESE SAUCE

This sauce is an ideal sauce for gluten-free pasta (hello, mac 'n' cheese!) or over vegetables, especially our Cauliflower "Rice" (page 163) or potatoes.

YIELD: About 1½ cups
PREP TIME: 10 minutes; **COOK TIME:** 10 minutes

½ cup nutritional yeast

2 tablespoons gluten-free flour (we like Bob's Red Mill version)

¼ teaspoon paprika

¼ teaspoon ginger powder

¼ teaspoon turmeric

2 tablespoons vegetable broth powder (try GoBIO! organic non-GMO yeast-free vegetable broth powder)

½ cup Almond Milk (page 148)

3 tablespoons tahini

1 tablespoon lemon juice

Optional: 1 pinch cayenne or chipotle pepper for more of a kick

Combine the nutritional yeast, flour, paprika, ginger powder, turmeric, and vegetable broth powder in a small saucepan and mix until combined.

Over medium-low heat, add the almond milk, ¼ cup of water, tahini, and lemon juice. Whisk until all the powder is dissolved and the sauce is smooth and thick, 2 to 4 minutes.

If the sauce is too thick, add more water to reach desired consistency. If too thin, add more nutritional yeast. Turn off the heat and season to taste.

SOUPS

These soups are perfectly healthy and balanced, but we exclude them from our core soup cleanses because of their whole animal protein, legumes, and/or grains, which, while excellent for your body, aren't so excellent when your digestive system is trying to get a much-needed break.

Spicy Shrimp and Coconut Soup

People who work out regularly or have a lot of muscle mass need more protein in order to sustain their bodies. This delicious and hearty soup with a little kick contains high levels of lean protein and vitamin and mineral content, and is one of the best ways to give your body what it needs and when it needs it. This isn't a soup we recommend for cleansing because of the shrimp, but it's a super-healthy option for everyday life.

YIELD: 6 servings
PREP TIME: 15 minutes; **COOK TIME:** 30 minutes

½ pound shrimp (not shelled)

1 lemon

1 onion, coarsely chopped

4 slices ginger or galangal

3 stalks lemongrass, tough husks removed, 2 thinly sliced, and 1 halved

4 garlic cloves, sliced

6 cups Roasted Vegetable Broth (page 143) or store-bought low-sodium
  (MSG-free, gluten-free) version

8 ounces flat rice noodles

1 tablespoon extra-virgin olive oil

2 medium shallots, sliced

3 Thai chilies, finely chopped (see note below)

1 red bell pepper, seeds and stem removed, cut into ½-inch slices

¼ cup fish sauce (can use a vegan version, if desired), plus more to taste

1 (14-ounce) can organic coconut milk (preferably Natural Value brand)

8 Thai basil leaves, sliced

Black pepper, to taste

½ bunch cilantro, coarsely chopped, for garnish

2 scallions, thinly sliced, for garnish

Thai Chilies

These very hot peppers add delicious heat to a dish and are rich in vitamins, minerals, and compounds that have antibacterial, anticarcinogenic, analgesic, and antidiabetic properties. But they can also burn the daylights out of your eyes if you're not careful. We recommend holding them by the stem (which you should discard) as you chop and then not touching the chopped chilies with bare hands.

First clean the shrimp by peeling off their shells (reserve these) and running a sharp knife down their backs. You'll see a thin brownish vein, which you can remove with the tip of your knife and your fingers. This is the shrimp's digestive tract—you don't want to eat it.

Place the cleaned shrimp in a bowl and zest the lemon over it. Toss to combine and place in the fridge.

Add the shrimp shells, onion, ginger, thinly sliced lemongrass, half of the garlic, and the vegetable broth to a medium-sized saucepan. Bring to a boil and then simmer for 15 minutes.

While the broth cooks, place the rice noodles in a medium-sized bowl filled with warm water and cover. The noodles should be done by the time the finished soup is, in approximately 30 minutes.

Strain the broth into a bowl and discard the solids. Set aside.

In the now-empty pan, add the olive oil and heat over medium-high heat until it dances. Add the rest of the garlic, shallots, and Thai chilies. Cook for 4 to 5 minutes. Add the red bell pepper and cook for 5 minutes or until the peppers are just beginning to soften.

Add the strained broth, fish sauce, and remaining lemongrass to the pot. Bring the soup to a boil, reduce to a simmer, and add the coconut milk. Be sure to keep the soup at a simmer from now on as boiling will cause it to separate.

Toss in the shrimp and Thai basil and cook until the shrimp are fully cooked, about 3 to 5 minutes. Taste and adjust the seasoning with fish sauce and pepper, if desired.

Strain the water from the rice noodles and divide the noodles among six soup bowls. Ladle the soup over the noodles and top with cilantro and scallions.

SPICY CHICKEN SOUP

While we don't advocate eating a lot of meat, having it in moderation—once or twice a week—is nourishing and balancing for the body. We've kept things from getting too heavy in this soup by combining the chicken with a deeply flavorful broth, brightened by chili sauce, vinegar, and lime. It's perfect for a weeknight dinner or to keep you going during a nonstop day. Just make sure you leave yourself a little time in advance to marinate the chicken.

YIELD: 4 to 6 servings
INACTIVE PREP TIME: 15 minutes to 1 hour;
  ACTIVE PREP TIME: 20 minutes; **COOK TIME:** 30 minutes

½ cup red wine vinegar

2 tablespoons red pepper flakes

3 skinless, boneless organic chicken breasts

2 tablespoons extra-virgin olive oil

4 garlic cloves, thinly sliced

2 medium shallots, thinly sliced

4 ounces (about ¼ cup) shiitake mushrooms, sliced

1 (1-inch) piece ginger, peeled and finely chopped

6 cups Chicken Broth (page 141) or store-bought low-sodium, gluten-free, (MSG-free, gluten-free) version

1 tablespoon fresh-squeezed lime juice

¼ cup fish sauce (substitute a vegan option, if desired)

1 small bunch (about ½ pound) baby bok choy, sliced

2 scallions, sliced, for garnish

1 lime, cut into 6 wedges, for garnish

First, make a Thai chili sauce by combining the red wine vinegar and red pepper flakes in a small bowl. Set aside for at least half an hour.

Place the chicken breasts on a cutting board. Notice that each has a "grain," or lines running through it. We recommend cutting against the grain, as it shortens the fibers in the chicken breast, creating a more tender slice. Slice the breasts into half-inch strips. We recommend starting at the small point of the breast and then turning it if necessary to keep slicing against the grain.

Transfer the slices of chicken to a small bowl and add 1 to 2 tablespoons of the chili sauce, enough to thoroughly coat the chicken. Let sit in the refrigerator for at least 15 minutes, but up to an hour is even better. Remove the chicken from the sauce to a paper towel.

In a medium-sized saucepan, heat 1 tablespoon of olive oil over medium-high heat until it begins to dance. Without crowding the pan, add the chicken strips. Allow them to brown, then use tongs to flip them over and brown the other side (about 1 to 2 minutes per side). You aren't cooking the chicken at this stage, just searing the outside to brown. You may need to do this in batches. If so, let the pan heat up after each new addition, adding more oil if necessary. Set the chicken aside.

Once all the chicken is seared and set aside, add another tablespoon of oil to the pot, along with the garlic, shallots, mushrooms, and ginger. Cook while stirring constantly, so the vegetables don't brown, about 2 minutes. Add the broth and bring it to a boil, then reduce to a simmer and cook for 10 more minutes.

Return the chicken to your saucepan and cook at a simmer until the chicken is fully cooked, 5 to 7 minutes. Add the lime juice, fish sauce, and bok choy and simmer just until the bok choy softens, about 2 minutes. Taste and adjust with salt, pepper, and chili sauce.

Serve with sliced scallions, lime wedges, and chili sauce. Any leftover sauce can last two to three days unrefrigerated or up to a month in the fridge in a covered jar.

CORN CHOWDER

As we said earlier, including a little non-GMO fresh, sweet corn from the farmers' market has its benefits, including its being an antioxidant and fiber-filled. So while it's not on our core soup cleanse, we do recommend this delicious, super-smooth and creamy non-dairy soup as one way to get those benefits in your regular diet.

YIELD: 4 to 6 servings
PREP TIME: 15 minutes; **COOK TIME:** 30 minutes

4 ears corn, kernels removed (about 4 cups) (see note below)

1 yellow or white onion, roughly chopped

3 garlic cloves, roughly chopped

½ cup Almond Milk (page 148)

3 carrots, chopped

2 golden beets, peeled and cubed

1 teaspoon ground cumin

1 teaspoon ground coriander

4 cups Chicken Broth (page 141), Roasted Vegetable Broth (page 143), or store-bought low-sodium (MSG-free, gluten-free) version

¾ cup coconut milk

Salt, to taste

Fresh cracked pepper, to taste

6 scallions, sliced (white and green parts)

The best method for removing corn kernels is to lay the cob flat on your cutting board and run your knife down the length of it. Rotate the cob, slicing kernels off with each turn.

Add 1 cup of corn kernels plus the onion, garlic, and almond milk to a blender and blend until smooth, 1 to 2 minutes.

Transfer the puree to a medium-sized pot and add the carrots, beets, cumin, coriander, remaining corn, and chicken broth. Bring to a boil then reduce to a simmer. Cook for 15 to 20 minutes, or until the carrots and beets are tender.

Stir in the coconut milk, making sure to keep the soup at a simmer so it doesn't separate. Season with salt and pepper, sprinkle in the scallions, and serve.

Dairy-Free New England Fish Chowder

For those seafood lovers who can't give up their creamy clam chowder, we have developed a non-dairy alternative—loaded with protein and iron—that will make you wonder what all the fuss over cream is in the first place.

YIELD: 4 to 6 servings
PREP TIME: 15 minutes; **COOK TIME:** 45 minutes

1 lobster tail
2 lemons
1 pound whole clams
1 tablespoon olive oil
4 garlic cloves, chopped
3 medium shallots, chopped
2 stalks celery, finely chopped
¼ teaspoon red pepper flakes
2 cups Roasted Vegetable Broth (page 143) or store-bought low-sodium
   (MSG-free, gluten-free) version
1 (8-ounce) bottle clam juice
3 parsnips, peeled and cubed
2 teaspoons dried thyme
1 tablespoon arrowroot powder
1 (8-ounce) can coconut milk
½ pound firm white fish like grouper, cod, or halibut, cut into 1-inch cubes
½ pound shrimp, cleaned and halved lengthwise
Salt and pepper, to taste

Clean the lobster tail by using kitchen shears (or well-cleaned scissors) to cut through the more delicate underside. Remove the lobster meat, chop it into 1-inch cubes, and place in a bowl. Set aside, reserving the tail shell.

Cut half of 1 lemon into slices and add to a large pot, along with the lobster shell, clams, and 2 cups of water. Bring to a boil and cook until the clams open, about 5 minutes. Remove the clams with tongs or a slotted spoon and transfer to a clean bowl, allowing the rest of the broth mixture to continue cooking. Remove the clam meat from the shells and return the shells to the pot once more. Cut each clam in half and set aside. Continue cooking the shells for 15 minutes.

Heat a medium-sized saucepan over medium-high heat and add the olive oil. When the oil dances, add the garlic, shallots, celery, and red pepper flakes. Cook, stirring, until the vegetables soften, about 5 minutes.

Using a colander or sieve, strain the homemade seafood broth into the pot with the garlic, shallots, and celery. Add the vegetable broth and clam juice and bring to a boil. Add the parsnips and thyme, reduce to a simmer, and cook for 5 minutes.

Add the arrowroot to a medium bowl. Take 1 cup of hot broth out with a measuring cup or ladle and slowly whisk it into the arrowroot until it dissolves and the broth thickens. Add the thickened mixture to the soup while stirring constantly until the soup begins to thicken.

Pour in the coconut milk along with the lobster meat, clams, fish, and shrimp and simmer until cooked, 4 to 8 minutes, depending on the size of your shrimp. Season to taste with juice from the remaining lemons, salt, and pepper.

BEEF BARLEY SOUP

Barley is a versatile grain that has a rich, nutty flavor and chewy, pasta-like texture. Its enormous dose of fiber is amazing for the digestive tract, sweeping out any unwanted visitors and feeding the friendly bacteria in the gut. Barley can also help lower cholesterol and prevent blood sugar levels from getting too high.[3] Though barley does contain gluten, it can be a beneficial addition to the diet if your body can handle it. Remember, we are all about balance. So while it is not part of our core soup cleanse, if your body welcomes it, barley is great in moderation. If not, simply substitute 1 cup of cooked brown rice, which has its own litany of health benefits, among them antioxidant protection, reducing blood sugar and blood pressure, decreased heart disease risk,[4] and fiber, fiber, fiber. Add in the deep, meaty flavor of beef shanks, and this soup is like a warm embrace on a cold winter's night.

YIELD: 8 to 10 servings
PREP TIME: 45 minutes; **COOK TIME:** 2½ hours

2 tablespoons extra-virgin olive oil

1 medium yellow onion, chopped

8 garlic cloves, chopped

2 stalks celery, chopped

3 carrots, sliced

3 pounds beef shanks

Salt and pepper, to taste

6 cups Richest Beef Bone Broth Ever (page 142) or store-bought low-sodium (MSG-free) version

2 bay leaves

1 bunch fresh thyme, tied with string

1 (14-ounce) BPA-free can or Tetra Pak whole tomatoes with juice

1½ cups barley, or 1 cup cooked brown rice

In a large saucepan, heat 1 tablespoon of olive oil over medium-high heat. When the oil dances, add the onion, garlic, celery, and carrots and cook for 5 minutes. Remove from the pan and add to a bowl. Set aside.

Add the remaining tablespoon of oil to the pan over medium-high heat. Season the shanks with salt and pepper and place in the pan. Brown on each side for 5 minutes. Remove the shanks to the same bowl as the vegetables.

Add 1 cup broth to the pan to loosen the browned bits on the bottom of the pan using a wooden spoon or whisk. Pour in the bowl of vegetables and beef, along with the bay leaves, thyme, remaining broth, and can of tomatoes. Bring to a boil, reduce to a simmer, and cook for 1½ hours.

Remove the shanks from the soup and transfer to a bowl. Set aside.

If using barley, add it to the soup, bring to a boil, and simmer for 30 to 45 minutes, or until the barley is tender but not mushy.

Remove any excess fat from the beef with your fingers and pull apart in smaller bite-sized pieces. Then return the beef pieces to the pot while the barley cooks. Season with salt and pepper to taste. If using brown rice instead, add it to the pot after the soup has cooked for 2 hours and allow it to simmer for about 10 minutes.

Note that the barley will absorb all the liquid if the soup isn't consumed immediately. If making this in advance to serve later, add additional broth when reheating.

LUNCH

GRILLED LEMON CHICKEN SALAD WITH MARKET GREENS AND CHERRY TOMATOES

With its vitamin C from antioxidant-rich lemons and mineral-bursting vegetables like leafy greens, cucumbers, and cherry tomatoes—high in iron, calcium, and magnesium—this bright, fresh salad is just the right hit of energy that won't leave you feeling overstuffed and undernourished. It's great for both lunch and dinner.

To save time, you can prepare the chicken ahead, up to one day before. Feel free to substitute salmon or grass-fed beef for the chicken.

YIELD: 2 servings
PREP TIME: 15 minutes; **COOK TIME:** Approximately 10 minutes

1 to 2 tablespoons extra-virgin olive oil
8 ounces boneless, skinless, organic free-range chicken breasts, cut into
   1-inch cubes
½ teaspoon sea salt
¼ teaspoon fresh ground pepper, plus more to taste
Juice of 1 lemon
1 tablespoon finely chopped fresh rosemary
2 cups fresh seasonal salad greens such as arugula, mesclun, kale, or
   spinach
½ cup sliced cucumbers, peeled
½ cup cherry tomatoes
1 to 2 tablespoons Lemon-Mustard Vinaigrette (page 163)

If using a grill: Preheat on medium-high heat.
   If using the oven: Preheat to 350°F.
   If using a pan: Heat 1 tablespoon of oil over medium-high heat.

Equipment: Metal or wooden skewers. Soak wooden skewers for 10 minutes before using.

Thread the chicken onto metal or wooden skewers. If using wooden skewers, be sure to soak them in water for 10 minutes to avoid burning them. Season with salt and pepper and grill for 6 to 8 minutes, turning halfway through; bake for 10 to 12 minutes, turning once or twice; or sauté for 6 to 8 minutes, turning halfway through. You know the chicken is done when the juices run clear.

In a medium bowl, whisk together the lemon juice, 1 tablespoon of olive oil, and rosemary. When the chicken is cooked, remove it from the skewers and toss it in the lemon juice mixture.

Arrange the salad greens on two plates. Top each serving with the sliced cucumbers, cherry tomatoes, and 4 ounces of lemon chicken. Drizzle 1 to 2 tablespoons of vinaigrette, season with freshly ground pepper, toss together, and enjoy.

SMASHED AVOCADO AND VEGGIE WRAP

(if using no-grain tortilla)
(if using raw tortilla or raw flatbread) Ⓡ

Mexican-inspired flavors make this otherwise simple vegetarian lunch a tantalizing treat. Who can resist the buttery taste of avocado with its silica-rich skin-boosting benefits? Pair it with iron-rich spinach and pH-balancing sea salt, and you've got a quick and tasty meal that will support you until snack time.

YIELD: 1 serving
PREP TIME: 10 minutes

¼ medium or ½ small avocado, flesh removed from skin
1 small gluten-free or raw tortilla or flatbread
Sprinkle of Himalayan pink salt or sea salt of choice, plus more to taste
Handful of baby spinach
¼ cup diced or sliced cucumbers
¼ cup shredded, slivered, or chopped carrots
Dash of cayenne pepper

Smash the avocado over the tortilla or flatbread. Sprinkle with salt and top with the veggies. Add a pinch more salt, if desired, and a dash of cayenne. Roll up the wrap and enjoy!

DINNER

BAKED WILD SALMON WITH AVOCADO, GINGER, AND MANGO SALSA

YIELD: 2 servings
PREP TIME: 10 minutes; **COOK TIME:** 15 to 20 minutes

4 teaspoons coconut oil
2 (3- to 4-ounce) wild-caught salmon fillets
Juice of 2 lemons
Optional: ½ teaspoon sea salt
Optional: ¼ teaspoon fresh cracked pepper
1 batch Avocado, Ginger, and Mango Salsa (recipe follows)

Preheat the oven to 325°F.

Grease the bottom of a baking sheet or oven-safe skillet with coconut oil. (Tip: You can also line a baking sheet with cookie parchment sheets—easy cleanup!) Drizzle both sides of the salmon fillets with the lemon juice and place them on the baking sheet or skillet. Sprinkle the fish with salt and pepper, if desired. Bake for 8 to 10 minutes on each side or until the fish is moist and flaky.

Top each piece of fish with a dollop of avocado, ginger, and mango salsa.

Avocado, Ginger, and Mango Salsa

½ cup mango (or papaya), diced into small cubes

1 avocado, diced into small cubes

1 red onion, minced

4 teaspoons finely chopped cilantro

½ teaspoon chopped fresh ginger (powdered works too!)

2 teaspoons seeded and minced jalapeño chili

½ teaspoon finely chopped fresh garlic

2 teaspoons fresh lime juice

In a medium bowl, mix the mango, avocado, onion, cilantro, ginger, chili, and fresh garlic. Sprinkle the lime juice over the salsa mixture and toss. Spoon the salsa on top of the baked fish. Serve and enjoy!

SESAME GARLIC CHICKEN AND BROCCOLI STIR-FRY OVER SIMPLE STEAMED BROWN RICE

(if omitting the rice)

This dish is enhanced with the flavors and healing benefits of Asian ingredients. There's calcium, fiber, minerals, and vitamins like B_1 from sesame seeds; vitamins A and C and iron from broccoli; and the anti-inflammatory effects of garlic and ginger. All in all, it's one immune-boosting feast.

YIELD: 2 servings
PREP TIME: 10 minutes; **COOK TIME:** 10 minutes

Sea salt

2 heads broccoli, stems removed, cut into 1-inch florets, or 3 cups frozen broccoli florets

2 tablespoons sesame oil

8 ounces organic boneless chicken, thinly sliced into 1- to 2-inch pieces

3 tablespoons freshly minced ginger

2 to 3 garlic cloves, minced

4 tablespoons wheat-free tamari or coconut aminos (a soy-free option)

Toasted sesame seeds, for garnish

Simple Steamed Brown Rice (recipe follows)

Bring 8 cups of water with a pinch of sea salt to a boil. Reduce to a simmer and add the broccoli. Cook until fork-tender, 2 to 3 minutes. Transfer from the water to a paper towel–lined plate and allow to cool.

Heat a wok or large sauté pan over medium-high heat and add the sesame oil. When it shimmers, carefully lay the chicken in the pan. Allow it to cook untouched for 1 minute before beginning to stir. After 3 minutes, add the ginger and garlic. Cook until just fragrant, then add the broccoli and tamari or coconut aminos.

Cover the pan with a lid and allow the mixture to cook for 2 to 3 minutes. Transfer to a large bowl and sprinkle with sesame seeds. Serve over brown rice.

Simple Steamed Brown Rice

Simple brown rice is simply full of fiber, and it's a great complement to our broccoli stir-fry. It's important that you buy organic brown rice, as conventional can contain high levels of arsenic.

YIELD: 2 servings
PREP TIME: 5 minutes; **COOK TIME:** 40 minutes

1 cup organic brown rice
Pinch sea salt

Use a strainer to rinse the rice of any debris. Put rice, salt, and 2 cups water in a pot with a tight-fitting lid. Bring to a boil, reduce to a simmer, and cover. Cook for 30 minutes. It's best to not lift the lid during that time. Instead, check the rice after 30 minutes and continue cooking for up to another 10 minutes if the water hasn't been fully absorbed. Fluff gently with a fork before serving.

BAKED HALIBUT WITH SWEET POTATOES AND SAUTÉED GREENS

Succulent halibut and nutrient-rich sweet potatoes, which are loaded with fiber and immune-boosting vitamin A, make this a hearty, comforting dish for everyone to enjoy. We've also included chlorophyll-powered greens that support energy, vitality, and daily cleansing.

YIELD: 2 servings
PREP TIME: 15 minutes; **COOK TIME:** 45 to 50 minutes

1 tablespoon extra-virgin olive oil or coconut oil, plus more for pan
8 ounces sweet potatoes or yams, peeled and cut into ½-inch-thick rounds
2 (4-ounce) halibut fillets (or other fish of choice)
Sea salt, to taste
1 to 2 shallots, thinly sliced
Pepper, to taste
Sautéed Greens (recipe follows)

Preheat the oven to 400°F. Lightly grease a 9-by-13-inch glass pan with olive oil. (You can also use a clay oven pot.)

Bring a medium pot of water to a boil and add the sweet potatoes. Boil for 10 to 15 minutes or until slightly soft.

Rinse the fish and pat dry with paper towels. Arrange the fillets in the pan so they sit in a single layer. Salt them on both sides. Top the fish with the sweet potatoes and shallots. Lightly drizzle the olive oil all over the ingredients and sprinkle pepper as desired. Bake for 35 minutes or until the fish is cooked through and the sweet potatoes are soft, tender, and ready to eat. Serve with the sautéed greens.

Sautéed Greens

These sweet chlorophyll-rich greens are loaded with immune-boosting garlic and lightly sprinkled sea salt for a flavor that's tasty and clean.

YIELD: 2 servings
PREP TIME: 10 minutes; **COOK TIME:** 5 minutes

2 teaspoons extra-virgin olive oil
2 cloves garlic, finely sliced
1 large or 2 small bunches kale, collard greens, or spinach, torn into small
   pieces
Sea salt and freshly ground pepper, to taste

Heat the olive oil in a medium to large skillet over medium heat. When warm, add the garlic and cook until soft, but not colored. Toss in the greens and let them cook until they are slightly wilted but still bright green, 3 to 5 minutes. Sprinkle with sea salt and pepper to taste.

SNACKS

Stave off the midmorning or afternoon energy slump with nutritious snacks that keep your metabolic fire burning, your mood balanced, and your belly happy.

Got the Munchies? Our Top Ten Snack Picks

Why is it that whenever we have the munchies, we head straight to the pantry or vending machine for chips, cookies, and other processed finger foods? It's usually because these foods are readily available and satisfy our immediate cravings for comfort, salt, and/or sweets. Make a commitment to skipping that vending machine and instead stocking your pantry and fridge with these tasty, on-the-go, nutritious snacks that won't make you break your commitment to good health.

And since we are talking about snack time after all, remember that fewer calories (especially as they relate to the right ratio of nutrients) are better. All you really need is a good, meaningful 100 calories to get you to your next meal. As we've said before, we don't advocate that you tally your caloric intake, but we do recommend that you are mindful of (a) how much food you need to feel satisfied, and (b) how full your calories are of nutrients (versus empty calories made from refined sugars and grains). We have done all the counting for you here with these on-the-go, nutritious treats packed with all the energy you need.

1. *No Nuts!: Dried Fava Beans*

For those with nut or gluten allergies, or for anyone else looking for an alternative to the basic handful of nuts, try fava beans roasted and dried. They're amazing for your nervous system and cellular function and are packed with folate, fiber, and iron. If you don't want to prepare them yourself, try Simply Beans' Fabz fava beans with sea salt. (If you want to roast your own fava beans, simply boil fresh fava beans in water for 20 to 30 minutes [until tender]. Drain the beans and toss them in olive oil [to lightly coat] and sea salt and pepper. Spread them, in a single layer, onto a baking sheet and roast at 375°F for about 25 minutes, but stir every 10 minutes to ensure even cooking.)

2. *Or, Go Nuts*

There really is no better snack nut, in our opinion, than almonds. They are loaded with protein and healthy fat, and studies have shown that eating them in moderation helps support heart health and prevent diabetes. If almonds just aren't your thing, try walnuts, Brazil nuts, or cashews. Or dress up your nuts with a teaspoon of dried cranberries. Make your own to-go bags by pre-measuring and storing in little snack bags.

3. Better Bitter Chocolate

If you can't escape that sweet craving, try dark chocolate, which is a powerful source of antioxidants, can improve blood flow and lower blood pressure, raises good cholesterol and lowers the bad, and may lower the risk of cardiovascular disease. Plus, it's just plain yummy. Aim for a version with 75 to 80 percent cacao.

4. Apples and Peanut Butter

Peanut butter sometimes just hits the spot. And if you buy the natural organic kind (without trans fats, palm oil, and refined sugar), it's a healthy snack too. Pair a couple of teaspoons with slices of apple for a magic combo of fiber, protein, and fat.

5. Edamame

Edamame, or boiled soybeans, are filled with protein and fiber, not to mention they are a delicious hot or cold snack all by themselves. Have ½ cup shelled or 1 cup still in the pod. Here's a little secret: If you eat them out of the shell, it will make the satisfying experience last much longer.

6. Strawberries with Whipped "Cream"

Pair 1 cup of fiber- and phytonutrient-rich strawberries with 2 tablespoons of homemade Whipped Coconut Milk (page 192) for a nutritious indulgence.

7. Raw Green Comfort (page 119)

Did we mention we love heart-healthy, potassium-rich avocados? Enjoy 4 ounces of this creamy, non-dairy "yogurt" soup for an afternoon or anytime snack.

8. *You Can Count on Cantaloupe*

Half a cantaloupe, our personal favorite of the melons, is not only filling (half of a melon is a whole lot of melon!), but it's also loaded with a wide variety of antioxidant and anti-inflammatory phyto-nutrients. No empty calories here!

9. *Calling All Egg Lovers!*

There's nothing much heartier (or easier) than a protein-packed egg for a snack. We love pairing them with fiber-full asparagus. Pair 10 spears (cooked or raw) with a hard-boiled egg and enjoy!

10. *Baby Carrots and Edamame "Hummus"*

You've never tasted hummus like ours, which uses miracle food edamame (recipe follows). Pair 4 teaspoons of it with celery sticks—or other crudités—and you've just packed in a ton of veggie power.

So-Delicious-I-Can't-Believe-It's-Green Dip, a.k.a. Edamame "Hummus"

This may be the tastiest—and healthiest—dip you have ever had with crudités, not to mention as a spread for sandwiches or sauce for gluten-free pasta. The edamame helps stabilize blood pressure and is attributed to helping with depression, while healing veggies and spices provide a host of vitamins and minerals. Tahini, a spread made from unhulled sesame seeds, is also an amazing superfood that has no shortage of benefits, including providing tons of calcium, preventing anemia, promoting healthy cell growth, packing more protein than most nuts, aiding liver detoxification, maintaining supple skin and muscle tone, and assisting in weight loss.

YIELD: 3 cups
PREP TIME: 15 minutes

2 tablespoons extra-virgin olive oil

½ cup fresh-squeezed lemon juice

2 tablespoons tahini

12 ounces shelled edamame (about 2 cups)

2 cups fresh baby spinach or baby arugula (packed down in cup)

⅓ cup flat-leaf parsley

2 tablespoons finely chopped yellow or white onion

3 medium garlic cloves

½ teaspoon cumin, plus more to taste

¼ teaspoon red chili or red pepper flakes, plus more to taste

1 teaspoon sea salt, plus more to taste

¼ teaspoon black ground pepper, plus more to taste

½ teaspoon poppy seeds, for garnish

1 teaspoon toasted sesame seeds, for garnish

Place the olive oil, lemon juice, tahini, edamame, spinach or arugula, parsley, onion, and garlic in a food processor or blender (a food processor works better than a blender for this). Blend on high for 1 to 2 minutes or until completely smooth (adding a tablespoon of water if the consistency gets too thick). Add the cumin, red chili or pepper flakes, salt, and pepper and blend to incorporate. Adjust seasoning if necessary to spice it up more.

Serve in a pretty bowl and sprinkle with poppy and toasted sesame seeds. Extra dip can be stored in an airtight container in the refrigerator for up to four days.

COCKTAILS

Sometimes a gal—or guy—just needs to get a little naughty. We're all about balance here at Soupure, and we too are only human. But if we are going to treat ourselves to a well-deserved cocktail, we're not going to skip the opportunity to work in some wellness too. We've taken some of our favorite infused waters and chilled soups and turned them into indulge-worthy treats.

BLUEBERRY MOJITO

Blueberries contain more antioxidants than almost all other fruits, vegetables, and spices, and studies show that they benefit the nervous system and brain health. In fact, there is new evidence that blueberries may improve memory. That's a pretty good case for throwing back one of these!

YIELD: 2 servings
PREP TIME: 5 to 10 minutes

4 sprigs fresh mint
1 cup Blueberry Mint Infused Water (page 115)
¼ cup fresh lime juice
6 tablespoons (3 ounces) bourbon
2 teaspoons organic agave
Ice

Place 2 sprigs of mint in a small bowl or cup and use the handle of a wooden spoon or a muddler to press into the leaves and twist. This will extract the mint flavor.

In a martini shaker or jar with a lid, combine the muddled mint, infused water, lime juice, bourbon, and agave with ice and shake. Pour into tall glasses filled halfway with ice. Use the remaining sprigs of mint to decorate each glass.

GREEN MARTINI

If you're going to have a cocktail, why not make it hydrating and healthy for the skin and body? Cucumber is rich in fisetin, which is crucial for brain health,[5] and it's otherwise full of potassium, magnesium, and fiber, making it balancing and soothing for the body. Honeydew is hydrating—essential for counteracting the effects of alcohol—while the dill pollen helps cleanse your liver, kidney, and spleen.

YIELD: 4 servings
PREP TIME: 5 to 10 minutes

¾ cup vodka
2¼ cups Cucumber-Grape-Honeydew Chilled Soup (page 116)
Ice
4 slices cucumber, for garnish
8 green grapes, for garnish
4 wooden or plastic sticks, for garnish

In a cocktail shaker or jar with a lid, combine the vodka, chilled soup, and a handful of ice and shake well (until very chilled). Pour into martini glasses.

Spear a slice of cucumber and 2 grapes on each skewer and place on the edge of each glass.

SUPER WHITE RUSSIAN

To make this take on a White Russian, you take our Superhero, the most nutrient-dense of all our soups, and add vodka and Kahlúa.

YIELD: 4 servings
PREP TIME: 5 to 10 minutes

½ cup vodka
1½ to 2 cups Superhero (page 151)
Ice

Combine the ingredients in a martini shaker or jar with a lid and shake until chilled. Pour into old-fashioned glasses over ice.

SWEETS

We like to think that even the saintliest saints have a sweet tooth, and that indulging in a little dessert every now and then isn't worth the guilt. Some sweet foods—especially high-quality chocolate, fruits, and natural sweeteners like honey and pure maple syrup—are actually beneficial to your health. Indulging in dessert is just another part of honoring healthy balance.

CHOCOLATE SOUP WITH SEA SALT ALMONDS AND WHIPPED COCONUT MILK

Chocolate may be considered a junk food, but semisweet and bittersweet chocolate have myriad health benefits—including lowering blood pressure, decreasing unhealthy cholesterol levels, and maintaining heart health[6]—with less sugar than milk chocolate. This dessert soup, in an otherwise healthy diet, offers a happy medium between satisfying that sweet tooth and adding health benefits.

YIELD: 3 to 5 servings
PREP TIME: 15 minutes; **COOK TIME:** 15 minutes

3 ounces high-quality bittersweet chocolate like Valrhona, roughly chopped

2 teaspoons arrowroot

2 cups Almond Milk (page 148)

1 cup coconut milk

1 teaspoon vanilla extract

1 tablespoon honey

1 batch Whipped Coconut Milk (page 192)

1 batch Sea Salt Almonds (recipe follows)

Optional: Organic pomegranate seeds, cranberries, or cherries

Fill a small saucepan with 1 inch of water and bring to a simmer. Add the chocolate to a medium heatproof bowl and set atop the pot to create a double boiler.

When the chocolate is almost completely melted with only a few solid pieces remaining, remove the bowl from the pot and stir to melt the remaining chocolate and smooth the mixture.

Add the arrowroot to a small saucepan and slowly pour in the almond milk while whisking to avoid lumps. Place the mixture over medium-low heat and continue whisking until the liquid thickens. Add the coconut milk, vanilla, and honey and whisk to incorporate. Slowly pour in the chocolate, stirring until it's completely combined. Remove from the heat, pour into bowls (it's rich—a little goes a long way!) with a dollop of whipped coconut milk and a sprinkle of sea salt almonds and, if desired, pomegranate seeds, and enjoy. If reheating the soup later, use the double-boiler method you used to melt the chocolate.

Sea Salt Almonds

Toasting almonds brings out their natural sweetness, accentuated by tossing them in sea salt. It's a sweet-and-salty combo that makes for an amazing snack or dessert garnish.

¼ cup whole raw almonds, coarsely chopped
1 teaspoon extra-virgin olive oil
1 teaspoon sea salt

Add the almonds to a small sauté pan and heat over medium heat. Cook while stirring constantly until the almonds are fragrant and browned, 7 to 10 minutes.

Over medium heat, pour in the olive oil and stir to coat the almonds. Sprinkle with sea salt and again toss to fully coat the nuts. Allow to cool and serve.

Whipped Coconut Milk

It doesn't get much more decadent than thick, creamy coconut milk whipped into a sweet topping.

1 small (5.6-ounce) can coconut milk, chilled overnight
1 teaspoon vanilla extract

For best results, place the bowl of an upright mixer or medium mixing bowl in the freezer for 5 minutes.

Skim the thick heavy cream off the top of the coconut milk and add to the chilled bowl. Add the vanilla and whip with a mixer or whisk until the milk thickens and forms semi-stiff peaks.

NUT PULP MACAROONS

YIELD: 14 to 16 macaroons
PREP TIME: 15 minutes; **COOK TIME:** 20 to 30 minutes

½ cup Medjool dates (or ½ cup maple syrup or agave syrup)
1 cup almond pulp (other pulps will work too; make sure all liquid is pressed out)
¼ teaspoon fine-grain salt
¼ cup oil (coconut oil tastes best)
¾ cup shredded coconut
1 tablespoon vanilla extract
Optional: ¼ teaspoon ground cinnamon

Preheat the oven to 350°F and line a baking sheet with parchment paper.

Combine the dates and nut pulp in a food processor and pulse to combine. Add the salt, oil, coconut, vanilla, and cinnamon, if using, and pulse until combined and uniform in texture. It's okay for it not to be completely smooth.

Using a tablespoon, scoop the batter onto the baking sheet. Bake for 20 to 30 minutes, checking regularly, until the macaroons are only lightly browned around the edges.

No-Cream Creamsicles

Hot summer day wearing you down? Kids clamoring for a sweet treat? Forget the ice-cream truck. Refresh with these richly rewarding veggie and fruit popsicles. Your body will thank you for it. The best part? You could use any of our chilled soups as bases.

Strawberry, Almond, and Chia Swirl Popsicles

YIELD: 4 to 6 popsicles
PREP TIME: 10 minutes; **FREEZE TIME:** 4 to 8 hours

2 cups strawberries, stems removed
1 tablespoon raw honey, maple syrup, or agave nectar
1 cup Almond Milk (page 148) or coconut milk
1 tablespoon chia seeds
½ tablespoon pure gluten-free vanilla extract

Blend the strawberries and ½ tablespoon honey, maple syrup, or agave until smooth, 1 to 2 minutes.

In a medium bowl, combine the almond or coconut milk and chia seeds, vanilla, and ½ tablespoon sweetener. Mix until combined.

Pour 1 to 2 tablespoons of strawberry puree into the bottom of each popsicle mold. Then, pour 1 to 2 tablespoons of the milk mixture. Alternate like this until the mold is full.

Chill in the freezer until completely frozen, 4 to 8 hours. To release the popsicles, try running the bottom of the molds under warm water for a few seconds—not too long because you want them loosened but not melted.

Pistachio and Banana Swirl Popsicles

YIELD: 4 to 6 popsicles
PREP TIME: 10 minutes; **FREEZE TIME:** 4 to 8 hours

1½ cups sliced bananas
1 tablespoon raw honey, maple syrup, or agave nectar
1 cup Pistachio Milk (page 150) or coconut milk
½ tablespoon pure vanilla extract

Blend the bananas and ½ tablespoon of honey, maple syrup, or agave in a blender until pureed, 1 to 2 minutes. Set aside.

In a medium bowl, combine the pistachio or coconut milk, vanilla, and ½ tablespoon of sweetener. Mix until combined.

Pour 1 to 2 tablespoons of banana puree into the bottom of each popsicle mold. Then pour in 1 to 2 tablespoons of the milk mixture. Alternate like this until the mold is full.

Chill in the freezer until completely frozen, 4 to 8 hours. To release the popsicles, try running the bottom of the molds under warm water for a few seconds—not too long as you don't want to melt the popsicles.

Avocado–Green Tea Popsicles

YIELD: 4 to 6 popsicles
PREP TIME: 10 minutes; **FREEZE TIME:** 4 to 8 hours

3 ripe avocados, halved, pitted, and flesh scooped out
1¾ cups organic coconut milk (Natural Value is our preferred brand)
1½ to 2 tablespoons agave nectar, to taste
½ tablespoon pure gluten-free vanilla extract
1½ tablespoons matcha powder

Add the avocado and coconut milk to a blender and blend until smooth, 1 to 2 minutes. You may need to further combine using a wooden spoon. Add the agave, vanilla, and matcha powder and blend until well combined.

Pour the mixture into molds* and freeze until completely frozen, 4 to 8 hours. To release the popsicles, try running the bottom of the molds under warm water for a few seconds, but not too long as you don't want to melt the popsicles.

* Note: Exposed areas will brown. To avoid, use covered molds.

Acknowledgments

There are many special people who have supported us along the whirlwind journey that led to the birth of this book. We extend our many thanks and gratitude to each and every one of you:

Our most dedicated employee, Kelsey De Gracia, who continues to give us hard work and inspirational guidance on our cleanse and nutrition and healing.

The many talented chefs who actually care about nutrition, health, and quality, beginning with Nicki Reiss and David Schlosser, continuing with Dale Greenblatt, and culminating with Joli Robinson. It is your input and recipe expertise that have made Soupure what it is today.

Our graphics and website manager, Brielle Hubert, who (with Lara Avila) has spent countless hours helping grow our business and making our "look" incredibly clean, modern, and sharp. And our social media expert, Lennisse Ambriz, for taking that look and helping us grow exponentially through the wacky world of social media.

Our medical team for their expertise and guidance, including Dr. Nada Milosavljevic, Dr. Farshid Rahbar, Dr. Charles Sophy, Dr. Harold Lancer, Dr. Whimsy Anderson, and Dr. Farshid Sam Rahbar. We cannot be more appreciative of the foreword written for us by Dr. Milosavljevic.

Our nutritionists, including Marlyn Diaz, who guide us and ensure our quality and sound nutrition, and Annie McRae and

Jennifer Cassada, who chant our praises and have been so supportive of our efforts to spread our word.

Richard Giorla, whose boundless enthusiasm, energy, and complete belief in Soupure keeps propelling us forward.

Michael and Michelle Chiklis, for believing in us from the very
first taste of our soups and whose love for the products led them to
being our first investors, our best customers, and our best supporters.

Our dedicated employees, who have stood with us, sharing the
growing pains along the way: Kelsey De Gracia, Joli Robinson, Rene
Banuelos, Oscar Sanchez, Chris Weinstein, Trever Noble, Brielle
Hubert, and Lara Avila.

Our literary agent, Meg Thompson, and our editor, Sarah Pelz, of
Grand Central Life & Style. You know we are sincere when we say we
would not be here without you both.

Photographer Victor Boghossian and Robin Tucker, our stylist,
who (assisted by our own Brielle Hubert) helped us create the beautiful photographs in this book.

Finally, our husbands, Daniel Blatteis and Nathan Hochman, for
your love and constant confidence and support that have carried us
on this amazing journey, and our children, Jacqlyn, Sabrina, and
Hudson Blatteis and Tyler, Harrison, and Brynn Hochman, who
have always supported us, believed in us, and have been willing to
try every soup no matter when, where, or what new ingredient we
decided to test!

Notes

Chapter 1: Getting Healthy in a Toxic World

1. "Chemical Body Burden," *Trade Secrets*, PBS, http://www.pbs.org /tradesecrets/problem/bodyburden.html.
2. Peter J. Delves, "Autoimmune Disorders," Merck Manual, http:// www.merckmanuals.com/home/immune-disorders/allergic -reactions-and-other-hypersensitivity-disorders/autoimmune -disorders.
3. Simone Reuter et al., "Oxidative Stress, Inflammation, and Cancer: How Are They Linked?" (2010), available at National Center for Biotechnology Information, http://www.ncbi.nlm.nih.gov/pmc /articles/PMC2990475/; V. Lobo et al., "Free Radicals, Antioxidants and Functional Foods: Impact on Human Health" (2010), available at National Center for Biotechnology Information, http://www.ncbi .nlm.nih.gov/pmc/articles/PMC3249911/.
4. "Research Sheds Light on Gluten Issues," Whole Grains Council, January 25, 2012, http://wholegrainscouncil.org/newsroom /blog/2012/01/research-sheds-light-on-gluten-issues.
5. "GMO Facts: Frequently Asked Questions," Non-GMO Project, http:// www.nongmoproject.org/learn-more/.
6. Dr. Amy Myers, "The Dangers of Dairy," Mindbodygreen, April 10, 2013, http://www.mindbodygreen.com/0-8646/the-dangers-of-dairy.html.
7. Steve Koenning and Gary Payne, "Mycotoxins in Corn," Plant Pathology Extension, North Carolina State University, http://www .ces.ncsu.edu/depts/pp/notes/Corn/corn001.htm.
8. Alice G. Walton, "WHO Says Monsanto Roundup Ingredient Is 'Probably Carcinogenic.' Are They Right?," *Forbes*, March 21,

2015, http://www.forbes.com/sites/alicegwalton/2015/03/21
/monsanto-herbicide-dubbed-probably-carcinogenic-by-world-health
-organization-are-they-right/.

9. R. F. Hurrell et al., "Soy Protein, Phytate, and Iron Absorption in
    Humans" (1992), available at National Center for Biotechnology
    Information, http://www.ncbi.nlm.nih.gov/pubmed/1503071; Sally
    Fallon and Mary G. Enig, "Newest Research on Why You Should
    Avoid Soy," Mercola.com, https://www.mercola.com/article/soy
    /avoid_soy.htm.

10. D. S. Bar-El and R. Reifen, "Soy as an Endocrine Disruptor: Cause
    for Action?" (2010), available at National Center for Biotechnology
    Information, http://www.ncbi.nlm.nih.gov/pubmed/21175082.

11. "Excess Sugar Linked to Cancer," *ScienceDaily*, February 1, 2013,
    http://www.sciencedaily.com/releases/2013/02/130201100149.htm.

12. "Artificial Sweeteners," Harvard T. H. Chan School of Public Health,
    http://www.hsph.harvard.edu/nutritionsource/healthy-drinks
    /artificial-sweeteners/.

13. "Review of *Excitotoxins: The Taste That Kills*," *Nutrition Digest* 37,
    no. 3 (1994), http://americannutritionassociation.org/newsletter
    /review-excitotoxins-taste-kills.

14. Dr. Thomas Rau and Susan Wyler, "Heart Disease: The Link Between
    Blood Acidity and Heart Disease," Biological Medicine Network,
    http://www.marioninstitute.org/biological-medicine-network
    /resources/articles/link-between-blood-acidity-and-heart-disease.

15. "How Does the Liver Work?," PubMed Health, November 22, 2015,
    http://www.ncbi.nlm.nih.gov/pubmedhealth/PMH0072577/.

16. Mae Chan, "Poor Diet Changes DNA, Causes Lasting Damage to
    Immune System," *Waking Times*, November 11, 2014, http://www
    .wakingtimes.com/2014/11/11/epigenetics-poor-diet-changes-dna
    -lasting-effects-immune-system/.

17. A. Gonzalez et al., "The Mind-Body-Microbial Connection" (2011),
    available at National Center for Biotechnology Information, http://
    www.ncbi.nlm.nih.gov/pubmed/21485746.

Chapter 3: The Soup Solution

1. Ian Sample, "Harvard Scientists Reverse the Ageing Process in
    Mice—Now for Humans," *Guardian*, November 28, 2010, http://
    www.theguardian.com/science/2010/nov/28/scientists-reverse
    -ageing-mice-humans; "Enzymes in Health and Disease," *Total*

Health, http://www.totalhealthmagazine.com/special-reports
/enzymes-in-health-and-disease.html.

2. Nancy Shute, "The Case Against Multivitamins Grows Stronger,"
Shots, National Public Radio, December 17, 2013, http://www.npr.org
/blogs/health/2013/12/17/251955878/the-case-against-multivitamins
-grows-stronger.

3. "Making Bone Broth a Staple in Your Diet May Be the Key to
Improving Your Health," Mercola.com, September 21, 2014, http://
articles.mercola.com/sites/articles/archive/2014/09/21/hilary
-boynton-mary-brackett-gaps-cookbook-interview.aspx.

4. "Raw vs. Cooked," Dr. Fuhrman, http://www.drfuhrman.com/faq
/question.aspx?qindex=4&sid=16.

Chapter 4: Your New Pantry Prescription

1. "Protein," Utah Department of Health/Women, Infants and
Children, http://health.utah.gov/wic/pdf/forms_and_modules
/Staff_Training_Modules/Basic%20Nutrition/basic%20nutrition%20
module%205.11_files/Page322.htm.

2. Vernon R. Young and Peter L. Pellett, "Plant Proteins in Relation
to Human Protein and Amino Acid Nutrition," *American Journal
of Clinical Nutrition* 59, no. 5 (May 1994), http://ajcn.nutrition.org
/content/59/5/1203S.long.

3. "Not Skin Deep: The Benefits of Organic Go Beyond the Peel,"
Organic Center, May 15, 2014, https://www.organic-center.org/news
/not-skin-deep-the-benefits-of-organic-go-beyond-the-peel/.

4. "GMO Foods Cause Gut Damage," Global Healing Center,
September 10, 2014, http://www.globalhealingcenter.com/natural
-health/gmo-foods-cause-gut-damage/.

5. Chris Keenan, "Top 10 Most Common GMO Foods," June 19, 2013,
http://www.cornucopia.org/2013/06/top-10-most-common-gmo-foods/.

6. "Is Carrageenan Safe?," DrWeil.com, http://www.drweil.com/drw/u
/QAA401181/Is-Carrageenan-Safe.html; Ann Daniels, "Xanthan Gum
Side Effects," LiveStrong.com, April 30, 2015, http://www.livestrong
.com/article/315249-xanthan-gum-side-effects/.

Chapter 6: Choosing and Preparing for Your Cleanse

1. Natural Resources Defense Council, "Smarter Living: Chemical
Index, Bisphenol A," December 28, 2011, http://www.nrdc.org/living
/chemicalindex/bisphenol-a.asp.

2. Bryan Walsh, "Study: Even 'BPA-Free' Plastics Leach Endocrine-Disrupting Chemicals," *Time*, March 8, 2011, http://science.time.com/2011/03/08/study-even-bpa-free-plastics-leach-endrocrine-disrupting-chemicals/.

Chapter 8: Cleansing Support: Moving, Breathing, and Sleeping

1. Michelle Castillo, "How Exercise Can Help You Ward Off Cancer," CBS News, August 20, 2013, http://www.cbsnews.com/news/how-exercise-can-help-you-ward-off-cancer/.
2. Marsha Anderson, "Four Easy Ways to Circulate Your Lymphatic Fluid," January 15, 2012, http://www.naturalnews.com/034649_lymphatic_fluid_rebounding_massage.html.
3. Robert Fraser et al., "Cortisol Effects on Body Mass, Blood Pressure, and Cholesterol in the General Population," *Hypertension* 33 (1999), http://hyper.ahajournals.org/content/33/6/1364.short.
4. Stanley Coren, "Are Dogs Trying to Communicate When They Yawn?," *Psychology Today*, April 25, 2012, https://www.psychologytoday.com/blog/canine-corner/201204/are-dogs-trying-communicate-when-they-yawn; "Scientists Aren't Exactly Sure Why We Yawn, but They Know Yawns Are Contagious," *Seed*, May 4, 2006, http://seedmagazine.com/content/article/the_incredible_communicable_yawn/.

Chapter 10: Core Cleanse Recipes

1. "An Avocado a Day May Help Keep Bad Cholesterol Away," American Heart Association, http://blog.heart.org/avocado-day-may-help-keep-bad-cholesterol-bay/.
2. "Daily Serving of Beans, Peas, Chickpeas or Lentils Can Significantly Reduce Bad Cholesterol," *ScienceDaily*, April 7, 2014, http://www.sciencedaily.com/releases/2014/04/140407122749.htm.
3. Michelle Raw, "Newest Study Reinforces the Prostate Cancer–Fighting Abilities of a Tomato-Rich Diet," August 29, 2014, http://www.naturalnews.com/046648_tomatoes_prostate_cancer_lycopene.html.
4. "Power Foods: Butternut Squash," *Whole Living*, http://www.wholeliving.com/134734/power-foods-butternut-squash.
5. "The Latest News About Green Peas and Broccoli," Mercola.com, April 29, 2013, http://articles.mercola.com/sites/articles/archive/2013/04/29/green-peas-broccoli-sprouts.aspx.

6. Elizabeth Renter, "Compound in Carrots—Falcarinol—Credited with Preventing Colon Cancer," Natural Society, June 9, 2013, http://naturalsociety.com/compound-falcarinol-carrots-prevent-colon-cancer/.

7. Melanie Grimes, "Eggplant Cures Skin Cancer," *Natural News*, November 17, 2009, http://www.naturalnews.com/027506_eggplant_skin_cancer.html.

8. Samantha Heller, MS, RD, "After-40 Nutrition: The Surprising Health Benefits of Beans," October 14, 2011, http://www.doctoroz.com/article/after-40-nutrition-surprising-health-benefits-beans.

9. "Bone Broth: How & 10 Reasons Why," Integrated Natural Medicine, http://www.integratednaturalmedicine.com/bone-broth/.

10. David Gutierrez, "The Secret Healing Benefits of Miso," July 30, 2012, http://www.naturalnews.com/036618_miso_fermented_food_nutrition.html.

Chapter 11: Healthy Pre-, Post-, and Mini-Cleanse Recipes

1. "3 Reasons to Eat Turmeric," DrWeil.com, http://www.drweil.com/drw/u/ART03001/Three-Reasons-to-Eat-Turmeric.html.

2. Mary-Jon Ludy and Richard D. Mattes, "The Effects of Hedonically Acceptable Red Pepper Doses on Thermogenesis and Appetite" (2011), available at National Center for Biotechnology Information, http://www.ncbi.nlm.nih.gov/pmc/articles/PMC3022968/.

3. "Dr. Perricone's No. 3 superfood: Barley," July, 15, 2005, http://www.oprah.com/health/Barley-Dr-Perricones-No-3-Superfood.

4. Marisa Ramiccio, "10 Surprising Health Benefits of Brown Rice," April 12, 2012, http://www.symptomfind.com/nutrition-supplements/brown-rice-health-benefits/.

5. Dr. Joseph Mercola, "9 Health Benefits of Cucumbers," August 23, 2014, http://articles.mercola.com/sites/articles/archive/2014/08/23/health-benefits-cucumbers.aspx.

6. Cleveland Clinic, "Heart Health Benefits of Chocolate," http://my.clevelandclinic.org/services/heart/prevention/nutrition/food-choices/benefits-of-chocolate.

Index

About the Authors

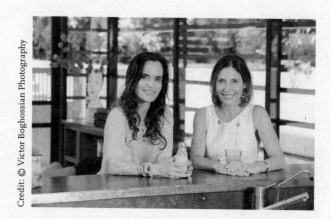

Credit: © Victor Boghossian Photography

ANGELA BLATTEIS (right) and VIVIENNE VELLA (left) founded Soupure to share the healing power of soups and souping. Both busy moms of three and hardworking professionals, Angela (from the world of private equity) and Vivienne (from the world of law) were perplexed by how challenging it was to find tasty, nutritious soups without cream or preservatives. So, they set out to create Soupure—a company that is in the business of developing and delivering nutrient-rich cold and hot soups, tonics and waters, and soup cleanses that are not only amazingly delicious and satisfying, but are also medically endorsed and made from organic, fiber- and protein-rich ingredients that are absolutely void of fillers and emulsifiers.